WALL PILATES FOR WOMEN OVER 40

A Journey to Enhanced Mobility and Strength to Transform Your Body with Gentle Movements

Carlos McDaniel

Table of Contents

Introduction

In the busy city of New Beginnings, tucked amid the lively cafés and bustling marketplaces, there was a little but beautiful bookshop famed for its selection of rare and life-changing books. Among its gems was a unique book called "The Wall Pilates Workout for Women Over 40: A Journey to Revitalized Strength and Grace."

The author of this guide, Sofia, is a Pilates instructor who is passionate about helping women regain their strength and energy through the discipline of Pilates. Sofia had seen a vacuum in the market for Pilates resources designed exclusively for women over 40. She noticed these women, like her friend Ava, struggle to find workouts that were appropriate for their needs—exercises that would build their bodies without risking injury, that would accommodate their hectic schedules, and that could be done in the comfort of their own home.

Sofia saw that the wall could be more than just a feature of the space; it could be converted into an instrument of empowerment. So she designed a guide that blended her Pilates experience with the wall's accessibility, allowing women anywhere to join in an effective and safe workout practice.

The book included 50 carefully selected activities, each of which was detailed and illustrated. These exercises were developed to promote not just physical strength, but also balance, flexibility, and overall well-being. From the "Wall Pike" to the "Wall Quad Stretch," each action was selected to provide a full-body workout that was both demanding and feasible for the over-40 audience.

However, "The Wall Pilates Workout for Women Over 40" was more than just an exercise handbook. It was a transformational story, matching the experiences of women like Ava who found hope in its pages. Women who had previously felt bound by their age were now embarking on a path of physical rejuvenation and self-discovery. They were enjoying exercise, improving their posture, and feeling stronger by the day.

Why should you purchase this guide? Because it is more than just a set of exercises. It is an invitation to join a community of women who are defying aging, recovering their power, and moving forward with fresh grace and confidence. It is for the lady who feels that her best years are not behind her but are taking place right now. It is for the woman who wants to invest in her health, who wants a practice that caters to her body's demands, and who appreciates the convenience of an exercise that can be done anywhere there is a wall.

Sofia's guide is more than simply a book; it's a partner on your path to a healthier, more vibrant you. It promises not only to improve your physique, but also to foster a deeper connection with oneself. In the busy metropolis of New Beginnings, among the numerous roads available, "The Wall Pilates Workout for Women Over 40" stands out as a light, directing women toward a future in which they feel powerful, energized, and unabashedly alive.

Overview of Wall Pilates

Wall Pilates, a refined version of conventional Pilates exercises, uses a basic vertical surface to improve workout efficacy and safety, making it an excellent training option for women over 40. This novel concept modifies Pilates exercises by leveraging the stability and resistance of a wall, giving support that aids in the maintenance of proper posture while executing various motions. It addresses typical concerns among women of this age group, such as the need for low-impact activities that lower the risk of injury while catering to a wide range of fitness levels.

Integrating the wall into Pilates workouts allows participants to engage more deeply with their core muscles, enhance their balance, and gain flexibility and strength in a regulated manner. This strategy allows for a progressive increase in intensity, guaranteeing that each individual may safely push herself without hurting her body. The tactile input from the wall also helps to increase body awareness, allowing users to alter their alignment and stimulate the appropriate muscle groups more efficiently.

Maintaining muscle mass and bone density is critical for women over 40's general health, and Wall Pilates helps them achieve both. Resistance-based workouts, such as wall squats and push-ups, promote muscular strength and endurance, which are essential for metabolic and bone health. Furthermore, focusing on core stability and strength aids in the relief and prevention of back pain, a common condition that can interfere with everyday activities and quality of life.

Flexibility and range of motion are two further areas where Wall Pilates excels, providing stretches and motions that are less daunting and more approachable than those found in typical Pilates or yoga courses. These motions are critical for preserving joint health, decreasing stiffness and discomfort associated with aging, and enhancing functional movements in daily life.

Furthermore, Wall Pilates emphasizes a mindful approach to exercise by urging participants to focus on their breathing and movement execution. This mindfulness practice can have a meditative impact, lowering stress and improving mental health. Such advantages are especially important for women over 40, who frequently manage several obligations and suffer the stress of midlife changes.

Participating in Wall Pilates courses or groups has a significant social impact. Joining a community of people who share your goals for better health and fitness may be extremely inspiring. It gives a sense of belonging and support, which is essential for sticking to a regular fitness regimen.

Finally, Wall Pilates provides a holistic training solution for women over 40, addressing both their physical and emotional health concerns. Its versatility, safety, and efficacy make it an appealing choice for individuals who want to keep their health, strength, and flexibility as they age. Women who incorporate Wall Pilates into their workout routine may have an active, balanced lifestyle with better physical abilities and a good view on their well-being.

Benefits of Pilates for Women Over 40

Pilates, particularly when modified to include the use of a wall, provides a distinct combination of strength, flexibility, and mindfulness that is ideal for the requirements of women over 40. Many women have a transitional period at this age, during which preserving bone density, muscle mass, and joint health becomes increasingly critical. Wall Pilates routines are designed to be low-impact, reducing the chance of injury while successfully addressing these vital regions. The wall's support helps women to do hard workouts with better control and accuracy. This greater control not only assures safety, but also enhances the efficacy of each exercise, resulting in better posture and core strength.

Women's metabolic rates and body composition frequently shift when they enter their forties. Wall Pilates programs address these changes front on by using a variety of aerobic and strength-training movements that can enhance metabolism and promote lean body mass. Wall Pilates' dynamic motions activate many muscle groups at once, making it an effective method to burn calories and improve strength without the need of heavy weights or high-impact aerobics. This makes wall Pilates especially appealing to people who want to manage their weight and keep their bodies toned as they become older.

The flexibility aspect of wall Pilates cannot be stressed. With aging, joints lose some of their range of motion, resulting in stiffness and diminished mobility. Wall Pilates movements gently urge the body to stretch and bend, with the wall serving as a support for deeper stretches and preventing overextension. This steady increase in flexibility leads to a more youthful, nimble physique that can conduct daily tasks with ease and is less prone to injury. Regular practice can result in considerable increases in overall flexibility, which can improve quality of life by making daily chores easier and less   unpleasant.

Wall Pilates movements also improve balance and coordination. As the body ages, keeping balance becomes more difficult, increasing the risk of falls and accompanying injuries. Wall Pilates develops the core and enhances proprioception, or the sensation of one's own posture, movement, and equilibrium, via targeted exercises that demand stability and control. These gains in balance and coordination are critical for avoiding falls, improving sports performance, and facilitating useful motions in everyday life.

Wall Pilates workouts provide both physical and mental health advantages. Pilates involves attention and awareness, transforming each session into a contemplative experience that can help with tension, anxiety, and sadness. The emphasis on breathing methods and the mind-body connection promotes a sense of serenity and well-being, making it an ideal practice for anyone dealing with the stressors and problems that frequently accompany midlife changes. This mental clarity and attention may be carried over into other aspects of life, increasing sleep quality, mood, and general mental   resilience.

Maintaining social connections and seeking out supportive groups might be critical for women over 40's general well-being. Participating in wall Pilates courses or groups allows you to meet others who have similar health and fitness objectives. This feeling of community may be extremely motivating, promoting frequent engagement and cultivating a shared sense of health and fitness. These organizations provide support and accountability, which may have a tremendous influence on one's dedication to living an active   lifestyle.

Wall Pilates provides a full workout that caters to the specific demands of women over 40. The benefits are numerous, ranging from increased physical strength, flexibility, and balance to better mental health and community ties. This type of exercise provides a long-term, low-impact alternative for preserving health and vitality well into midlife and beyond, making it a crucial tool for women looking to age gracefully and healthily.

How to Use This Guide

Starting the Wall Pilates journey for women over 40 entails adopting a one-of-a-kind and revolutionary approach to exercise that combines Pilates principles with the supporting help of a wall. This book is precisely developed to meet the special demands of women in this age group, recognizing the intricacies of their physical condition and the need of a regimen that strengthens, tones, and increases flexibility without putting excessive strain on the body. The key benefit of utilizing this book is its capacity to adapt to individual fitness levels, providing a choice of workouts ranging from beginning to expert, guaranteeing a smooth and safe improvement in strength and technique.

This guide is built on the principle of mindful movement. Each exercise is intended to not only increase physical strength and flexibility, but also to build a strong bond between mind and body. The guide encourages practitioners to build inner serenity and balance by stressing controlled, precise movements as well as the importance of breathwork. This attentive technique is especially good for women over 40 since it reduces stress, improves mental clarity, and boosts general well-being.

The tutorial explains the notion of using the wall as a workout companion rather than a prop. The wall provides resistance, support, and feedback, allowing you to fine-tune your alignment and execution for each exercise. Whether performing squats, stretches, or more difficult Pilates routines, the wall helps to achieve proper form, boosting workout efficacy and lowering the chance of injury. This creative use of the wall makes Pilates more accessible and pleasant, allowing a wide range of exercises to be safely practiced at home.

Flexibility in the training program is another important part of this strategy. Understanding that women over 40 typically have several commitments, the book is designed to fit effortlessly into a variety of schedules. Exercises may be combined to create shorter or longer exercises based on available time, making consistency simpler to maintain. This adaptability ensures that being healthy does not become a cause of stress, but rather a refreshing respite from the responsibilities of daily life.

To ensure that practitioners get the most out of their Wall Pilates exercises, the book stresses establishing realistic objectives and listening to their bodies. It encourages women to approach their fitness journey with patience and care, gradually increasing strength and flexibility without pushing their bodies to their limitations. This empathetic approach is essential for developing a sustainable and pleasurable workout regimen that can be maintained over time.

The integration of the exercises into daily life is a key element of the handbook. Aside from planned workouts, it provides methods to use Pilates concepts in everyday tasks. This comprehensive approach guarantees that the exercises' effects last beyond the workout sessions, resulting in improved posture, enhanced core strength, and better movement patterns in everyday life. It is about developing a lifestyle that embraces Pilates ideals while boosting health   and   energy.

Finally, this book provides a thorough resource for ladies over the age of 40 who want to start doing Wall Pilates. With its emphasis on conscious movement, adaptation, support, and overall well-being, it provides a method for building physical and mental strength that is both effective and loving. Practitioners who follow the guidance may expect to not only alter their bodies but also improve their overall quality of life, demonstrating that age is just a number when it comes to embracing health and fitness.

Getting Started

Preparing Your Space

Creating an appealing and efficient area for wall Pilates routines, particularly for ladies over 40, begin with selecting the appropriate wall. This wall should be strong and clear of impediments, giving a stable foundation for workouts that improve strength, flexibility, and balance. The ideal wall is smooth and clean, free of artwork, decorations, and anything that might impede movement or cause damage. It is critical to have adequate space to move freely, therefore keep a clean area surrounding the wall. This area does not have to be big, but it should be adequate to allow for complete range of motion in all directions.

Lighting in your Pilates studio is essential for establishing a welcoming environment that encourages frequent practice. Natural light is extremely useful, fostering a sense of well-being and aiding concentration during exercise. If natural light is not available, soft, artificial lighting that uniformly lights the room without causing glare or shadows can be used to provide a comfortable environment for your workout. The idea is to have enough light to see properly but not so bright that it causes pain.

Another important factor to consider is the surface on which you exercise. A yoga or Pilates mat offers padding and grip, ensuring comfort and stability when practicing movements against a wall.

The mat should be thick enough to support your spine during floor movements while also providing a sturdy platform for standing and sitting poses. Placing the mat perpendicular to the wall enables for a smooth transition between workouts requiring wall assistance and those performed on the floor.

Temperature and ventilation are important elements in determining comfort and endurance during an exercise. To avoid muscular stiffness or overheating, keep the environment at a suitable temperature that is neither too hot nor too cold. Good ventilation is also required to guarantee fresh air circulation, which helps to retain energy and attention during the Pilates practice. If the room is stuffy, a fan or an open window might offer enough air movement to improve the entire workout experience.

Personalizing the area may significantly boost motivation and satisfaction. Adding inspirational items, such as encouraging phrases, relaxing colors, or a tiny plant, can help to create a nice and inspiring workplace. To prevent distractions, keep things simple. The emphasis should be on providing a peaceful environment that promotes concentration and awareness during the Pilates session.

When preparing your area for Pilates, make safety a top consideration. Check that the floor is not slippery and that the area surrounding the wall is free of dangers that might cause trips or falls. It's also a good idea to keep a water bottle on hand to stay hydrated, as well as a towel to wipe away sweat. These practical factors can help you have a safe and uninterrupted training session.

Finally, using technology wisely may improve your Pilates practice. A mirror positioned opposite the wall can aid in checking form and technique, while a speaker playing quiet music can provide a relaxing rhythm for the workout. If you're taking online classes or tutorials, ensure sure your gadget is positioned so it can be easily viewed without straining your neck. This setting promotes a holistic approach to wall Pilates by establishing a place that is both functional and loving, encouraging women over 40 to practice Pilates on a regular basis with confidence and ease.

Safety Tips

Starting from a wall Pilates training program provides a unique combination of strength, flexibility, and balance exercises intended for women over 40, but it is critical to begin this fitness routine with caution. First and foremost, ensuring that the physical environment is ready can significantly lower the risk of damage. A clean location with a robust, smooth wall free of barriers is required to do exercises without slipping or bumping into anything. A safe training setting should also have adequate lighting and a non-slip mat, which provide visibility and stability during each activity.

Before beginning any wall Pilates sequence, it is critical to check one's health status, especially if you are new to training or have pre-existing health problems. Consulting with a healthcare practitioner might offer information on any limits or precautions that should be taken. This professional assistance is crucial because it assures that the activities chosen will be both effective and safe, taking into account particular health concerns.

Warm-up activities are essential for getting the body ready for the activity ahead. A simple sequence of stretches and mobility exercises can assist to enhance blood flow to the muscles, reduce stiffness, and lower the chance of injury. Incorporating a warm-up that particularly targets the muscles and joints to be utilized in the wall Pilates session will help to smooth and improve the transition to more intense movements.

Understanding the proper form and technique for each exercise is another critical safety precaution. Wall Pilates, like any other kind of exercise, necessitates accuracy to maximize the benefits of each action while reducing the danger of strain or injury. Learning the proper posture and motions from a trained Pilates teacher or from trusted internet materials will help you practice wall Pilates safely.

Women over the age of 40 who do wall Pilates must pay attention to their bodies' cues during the workout. The body's response to exercise might change from day to day, and what was manageable in one session may feel more difficult in another. It is critical to recognize these signals and alter the intensity of the workout properly to avoid overexertion, which can lead to injury.

Rest and water are equally as crucial as the activities themselves. Taking pauses as appropriate assists the body to recuperate, particularly during longer or more severe workouts. Staying hydrated aids in muscle function and cramp prevention, making for a safer and more successful workout.

Finally, the necessity of cooling down cannot be overstated. Just as the body needs to prepare for a workout, it also needs time to recover afterwards. A cool-down session involving stretches and moderate movements helps to gradually lower heart rate, avoid muscular discomfort, and improve flexibility. This last element of the exercise is critical in providing a thorough and safe wall Pilates experience, laying the groundwork for recuperation and preparation for the next session.

Warm-Up Exercises

Warm-up activities are essential for getting the body ready for a wall Pilates session, especially for women over 40. These early motions assist to enhance blood flow to the muscles, slightly raise the heart rate, and gradually stretch the muscles, making them more flexible and less prone to injury. Beginning a wall Pilates session with a series of mild stretches against the wall may successfully target major muscle groups while also providing the stability required by older persons or those with balance issues.

Engaging in wall arm slides is an efficient technique to get started. This exercise helps to release the shoulders and upper back, which are regions where tension can build. Participants stand with their back flat against the wall, gently sliding their arms up above and then back down, maintaining their arms and back in touch with the wall the entire time. This action not only warms up the shoulders, but it also promotes good posture by engaging the core muscles.

Another warm-up action is to perform modified leg swings against the wall. By holding onto the wall for support, one may gently swing one leg forward and backward before switching to side-to-side movements. This warms up the hip joints, hamstrings, and quadriceps, getting the legs ready for exercises like wall squats and leg lifts, which are typical in Pilates workouts.

Wall push-ups are a great technique to warm up the chest, arms, and core before moving on to more difficult workouts. Beginning with hands on the wall at shoulder height and feet a reasonable distance apart, bend the elbows to bring the chest closer to the wall before pushing back to the beginning position. This exercise activates the upper body and core, preparing them for the activity ahead.

A wall-supported cat-cow stretch can help improve flexibility and prepare the spine for Pilates techniques. With hands on the wall at waist height, arch the back upward, tucking the chin into the chest, then reverse the curve, elevating the head and tailbone. This is similar to the typical cat-cow yoga stance, but the wall provides additional support and a softer stretch.

Incorporating a wall sit into your warm-up regimen will assist stimulate your lower body, especially your thighs and gluts. Sliding down the wall to a sitting posture, thighs parallel to the floor, and holding for several seconds strengthens the legs and increases endurance. It's a simple yet effective approach to get your muscles ready for Pilates movements that need lower-body strength and stability.

Finally, ending the warm-up with deep breathing exercises against the wall will help center the mind and body, establishing a calm and concentrated tone for the Pilates practice. Standing with your back against the wall and taking deep, calm breaths helps to oxygenate and relax the muscles. This exercise not only warms up the physical body but also prepares the mind, resulting in a balanced start to the Pilates session.

Core Strengthening Exercises

Wall Pike

The Wall Pike is a dynamic and effective core strengthening exercise within the realm of Wall Pilates, particularly beneficial for women over 40. This exercise not only targets the abdominal muscles but also engages the shoulders, arms, and hamstrings, offering a comprehensive workout that enhances overall stability and core strength.

Instructions for Performing the Wall Pike:

1. Start in a standing position facing away from the wall. Walk your feet towards the wall and place your hands on the floor, ensuring they are shoulder-width apart.

2. Walk your feet up the wall until your body forms an inverted "V" shape. Your hands should remain flat on the floor, directly under your shoulders. Your legs and arms should be straight, with your heels gently pressing against the wall.

3. Engage your core muscles by drawing your navel towards your spine. This engagement is crucial for stability and effectiveness.

4. From this position, slowly push through your arms and shoulders, elevating your hips even higher towards the ceiling. The movement should be controlled and driven by the strength of your core.

5. Hold the peak position for a few seconds, focusing on the contraction in your abdominal muscles.

6. Carefully lower your hips back to the starting inverted "V" position without losing the tightness in your core or the straightness of your legs and arms.

7. Repeat the exercise for several repetitions, according to your comfort and fitness level.

Benefits of the Wall Pike:

- Enhances Core Strength: The Wall Pike exercise specifically targets the abdominal muscles, including the rectus abdominis and the deeper core muscles like the transverse abdominis. This leads to improved core stability, which is essential for balance and overall body strength.

- Improves Shoulder Stability: By engaging the shoulders and arms, this exercise also helps to strengthen the upper body, contributing to better posture and reducing the risk of shoulder injuries.

- Increases Flexibility in Hamstrings: The inverted "V" position stretches the hamstrings, which can help alleviate stiffness and improve flexibility in the lower body.

- Promotes Balance and Coordination: Performing the Wall Pike requires and enhances balance and coordination, as it involves maintaining a controlled position against the wall.

- Suitable for Varying Fitness Levels: Although challenging, the Wall Pike can be modified to suit different fitness levels. Beginners can start with a lower elevation of the hips, gradually increasing as strength and confidence build.

Wall Teaser

The Wall Teaser is a dynamic exercise within the realm of Pilates that specifically targets the core, enhancing strength, stability, and balance. For women over 40, incorporating the Wall Teaser into their Wall Pilates workout offers numerous benefits, including improved posture, enhanced core strength, and a reduction in lower back pain. This exercise adapts the traditional Pilates Teaser to use the wall as a form of support, making it more accessible and providing a way to focus on form and alignment.

To perform the Wall Teaser, follow these instructions:

1. Begin by sitting on the floor with your legs extended straight in front of you and your back against the wall. Ensure your spine is aligned with the wall from your tailbone to your head.

2. Extend your arms overhead, keeping them straight and parallel to your ears. Your hands should lightly touch the wall above you.

3. Inhale to prepare, engaging your core muscles.

4. As you exhale, slowly start to peel your spine off the wall, vertebra by vertebra, lifting your arms and torso up towards your toes. Your legs remain straight and grounded.

5. Inhale as you pause at the top of the movement when your body forms a "V" shape.

6. Exhale and slowly roll your spine back down to the starting position against the wall, maintaining control and alignment.

The benefits of the Wall Teaser for women over 40 are significant. Firstly, it strengthens the core muscles, including the abdominals, back, and pelvic muscles, which are crucial for maintaining good posture and reducing the risk of back pain. Strengthening these muscles through exercises like the Wall Teaser can also improve overall stability and balance, reducing the risk of falls. Additionally, the controlled movement required to perform the Wall Teaser enhances flexibility in the spine and promotes a greater range of motion. This exercise also encourages mindful movement and concentration, as focusing on the breath and the precise alignment of the body can have a calming effect on the mind.

Wall Roll-Up

The "Wall Roll-Up" is a pivotal exercise in the Wall Pilates workout, especially beneficial for women over 40 seeking to strengthen their core muscles. This exercise is an adaptation of the classic Pilates roll-up, utilizing the wall to provide additional support and feedback for the movement. The Wall Roll-Up targets the abdominal muscles, promotes spinal flexibility, and enhances control over the body's core. Its effectiveness lies in the smooth, controlled motion that challenges the core throughout the range of movement.

To perform the Wall Roll-Up:

1. Begin by sitting on the floor with your legs extended straight in front of you and your feet flat against the wall. Ensure there's a small gap between your feet and the wall for movement flexibility.
2. Lean back slightly, placing your hands on the mat behind your hips for initial support. Engage your abdominal muscles to prepare for the movement.
3. Slowly roll down onto your back, vertebra by vertebra, allowing your arms to extend overhead towards the floor. The back of your hands may lightly touch the ground at the lowest point.
4. Inhale deeply, and as you exhale, reverse the movement. Engage your core to lift your arms overhead, leading with

your fingertips towards the wall. Peel your spine off the mat, articulating each vertebra as you come up.

5. As your hands reach the wall, use the slight resistance to help stretch further, elongating your spine and reaching forward with your hands. Maintain engagement in your abdominal muscles to control the movement.

6. Inhale as you prepare to roll down again, and repeat the exercise for the desired number of repetitions.

The benefits of the Wall Roll-Up for women over 40 are significant:

- Core Strengthening: This exercise deeply engages the abdominal muscles, including the transverse abdominis, rectus abdominis, and the obliques, leading to improved core strength and stability. A strong core is crucial for overall body strength, balance, and preventing lower back pain.
- Spinal Flexibility: The articulation of the spine during the roll-up and roll-down phases promotes greater spinal mobility. This can help alleviate stiffness and promote a healthier, more flexible spine, which is particularly important as flexibility tends to decrease with age.
- Improved Posture: By strengthening the core and enhancing spinal flexibility, the Wall Roll-Up can contribute to better posture. Good posture is essential for

reducing the strain on the spine and preventing the onset of back pain.

- Enhanced Body Control and Awareness: Performing the Wall Roll-Up requires concentration and control, fostering a heightened sense of body awareness. This can translate into improved coordination and balance, reducing the risk of falls and injuries.
- Breath Control: The synchronized breathing pattern required for this exercise helps improve lung capacity and oxygenation, and it also supports the meditative aspect of Pilates, promoting relaxation and stress relief.

Wall Roll-Down

The "Wall Roll-Down" is a fundamental exercise within the Wall Pilates Workout, especially beneficial for women over 40. This core-strengthening exercise focuses on the spine's articulation, engaging the abdominal muscles deeply, and enhancing flexibility in the back. Its simplicity and effectiveness make it a staple in Pilates routines, providing a gentle yet impactful way to warm up the body and prepare for more intensive exercises.

Instructions:

1. Start by standing with your back against a wall, feet hip-width apart and slightly away from the base. Your heels should be a few inches from the wall, aligning your body in a straight posture from head to heels.
2. Inhale deeply, filling your lungs and preparing your body for movement.
3. As you exhale, begin to tuck your chin to your chest, allowing your head to start the motion of rolling down. The objective is to peel your spine off the wall vertebra by vertebra, starting from the neck and moving downwards.
4. Continue rolling down as far as comfortable, aiming to reach towards your toes. It's not about touching your toes but rather feeling a stretch along your spine and engaging your core muscles.
5. Pause at the lowest point of your roll-down for a breath, keeping your abdominal muscles engaged.

6. Inhale and start rolling back up against the wall. Imagine restacking each vertebra against the wall, from your lower back up to your neck, ending with your head coming up last to return to the starting position.

Benefits:

The Wall Roll-Down is particularly advantageous for women over 40 for several reasons. Firstly, it encourages spinal flexibility, which can decrease with age. By actively engaging in exercises that promote spinal articulation, women can help maintain a healthier, more flexible spine, reducing the risk of stiffness and pain that can accompany aging.

Secondly, this exercise deeply engages the core muscles, including the transverse abdominis, which are crucial for overall stability and strength. Strengthening these muscles contributes to better posture, reduced lower back pain, and improved balance, which are essential for daily activities and overall health.

Additionally, the Wall Roll-Down serves as a mindful exercise that encourages body awareness. Performing the exercise slowly allows women to tune into their bodies, noticing areas of tension and practicing control over their movements. This heightened awareness can improve the effectiveness of their Pilates practice and contribute to a greater sense of well-being.

Moreover, the wall provides feedback on the movement, ensuring proper alignment and helping to prevent injury. This aspect is particularly beneficial for beginners or those who may have concerns about executing exercises correctly.

Wall Plank

The Wall Plank is a core strengthening exercise that has been adapted for the Wall Pilates Workout, particularly beneficial for women over 40. This variation of the traditional plank exercise uses the wall as a support, making it more accessible and reducing the strain on the lower back and shoulders, areas where women in this age group may have concerns. The wall plank focuses on engaging and strengthening the core muscles, including the abdominals, back muscles, and obliques, while also offering stability and support.

Instructions for Performing a Wall Plank:

1. Start by standing facing the wall, approximately an arm's length away.
2. Place your hands on the wall at shoulder height, keeping them shoulder-width apart.
3. Walk your feet back until your body is at a slight incline, forming a straight line from your head to your heels. Your arms should be straight, supporting your body weight.
4. Engage your core muscles by drawing your belly button towards your spine and tightening your abdominal muscles. Ensure your body remains in a straight line without sagging or arching your back.
5. Hold this position, focusing on keeping your core engaged and breathing steadily. Aim to maintain the plank for 20-

30 seconds to start, gradually increasing the duration as your strength improves.

6. To end the exercise, slowly walk your feet forward, returning to a standing position.

Benefits of the Wall Plank:

- Improved Core Strength: Regular practice of the wall plank strengthens the core muscles, which is crucial for overall stability, balance, and posture.

- Enhanced Postural Support: Strengthening the core muscles through exercises like the wall plank can lead to better posture, reducing the risk of back pain commonly experienced by women over 40.

- Increased Balance and Stability: A strong core enhances balance and stability, which can help prevent falls and improve performance in daily activities as well as other physical exercises.

- Accessibility: The wall plank is a low-impact exercise that is accessible to women over 40, regardless of their fitness level. It can be modified by adjusting the distance of the feet from the wall to increase or decrease the intensity.

- Reduction in Lower Back Pain: By strengthening the core, the wall plank can help alleviate lower back pain, a common issue for many women in this age group. A strong core takes pressure off the lower back, supporting the spine.

- Versatility: This exercise can be easily incorporated into any workout routine and requires no special equipment, making it perfect for home workouts.

Wall Bicycle

The "Wall Bicycle" is a dynamic exercise within the Wall Pilates workout regime, particularly beneficial for women over 40 seeking to enhance their core strength, improve their abdominal muscle tone, and increase the flexibility of their lower back and hips. This exercise, adapted from the traditional floor bicycle crunch, uses the wall as a prop to add an extra stability challenge, making it an innovative way to engage the core muscles more effectively while minimizing strain on the back.

To perform the Wall Bicycle, follow these instructions:

1. Begin by lying on your back a short distance from the wall, with your legs extended upwards and your feet placed flat against the wall, creating a 90-degree angle with your body.
2. Place your hands behind your head, keeping your elbows wide to open up the chest.
3. Engage your core by drawing your belly button towards your spine and lift your shoulders slightly off the ground to enter the starting position.
4. Now, simulate the pedaling motion by bending one knee and bringing it towards your chest while extending the other leg, keeping both feet against the wall.

5. As you 'pedal,' rotate your torso so that the opposite elbow moves towards the knee that is bending towards your chest.

6. Alternate sides in a smooth, controlled manner, ensuring that you maintain core engagement and controlled breathing throughout the exercise.

The benefits of the Wall Bicycle for women over 40 are manifold:

- Core Strengthening: This exercise targets the rectus abdominis, obliques, and the transverse abdominis, helping to build a stronger, more stable core.
- Reduced Back Strain: Performing the bicycle movement against the wall provides lower back support, reducing the risk of strain compared to traditional floor crunches.
- Increased Flexibility: The rotational movement enhances flexibility in the spine, contributing to better mobility and reducing the risk of back pain.
- Improved Balance and Stability: By using the wall for support, this exercise challenges your balance and stability, key components in preventing falls and maintaining functional mobility.
- Enhanced Coordination: The cross-body movement pattern of the Wall Bicycle encourages better coordination and neural connectivity between the left and right hemispheres of the brain.

Wall V-Sit

The Wall V-Sit is a dynamic core strengthening exercise that holds particular benefits for women over 40 engaging in a Wall Pilates Workout. This exercise not only targets the abdominal muscles but also engages the deeper core muscles, which are essential for improving posture, enhancing balance, and reducing the risk of back pain. The support of the wall in this Pilates exercise adds an element of stability, making it more accessible for individuals at different fitness levels while still offering the challenge needed to strengthen the core effectively.

Instructions for performing the Wall V-Sit:

1. Start by sitting on the floor with your legs extended in front of you and your back against the wall. Your body should form a straight line from your head to your heels, with your hands on the floor beside your hips for support.

2. Engage your core muscles and lift your legs off the floor, pressing your back firmly against the wall. For beginners, a slight bend in the knees can help maintain form without straining the lower back.

3. Extend your arms forward parallel to the floor, keeping your shoulders down and away from your ears to maintain a long, neutral neck.

4. Lean back slightly at the hips while keeping your back straight and press against the wall. Lift your legs higher to

form a V shape with your body. The sharper the angle, the more challenging the exercise will be.

5. Hold this position for a few seconds, focusing on keeping your core engaged and breathing steadily.

6. Slowly lower your legs back to the starting position and repeat the exercise for several repetitions, according to your fitness level and comfort.

Benefits of the Wall V-Sit in a Wall Pilates Workout for Women Over 40 include:

- Core Strengthening: This exercise intensely targets the abdominal muscles, including the rectus abdominis, obliques, and the deep transverse abdominis, which support the spine and improve overall stability.

- Improved Posture: Strengthening the core muscles helps in maintaining an upright posture, which can often be compromised with age due to muscle weakness and imbalances.

- Enhanced Balance and Stability: By engaging the core muscles, the Wall V-Sit helps improve balance and stability, which are crucial for preventing falls and maintaining independence as we age.

- Increased Flexibility: The action of maintaining the V position encourages flexibility in the hamstrings and lower back, areas where women over 40 often experience tightness.

- **Low Impact:** Using the wall for support makes this exercise low impact, reducing strain on the joints and making it suitable for those with knee or hip concerns.

Upper Body Exercises

Wall Push-Up

The Wall Push-Up is a fundamental exercise in the Wall Pilates Workout, especially designed for women over 40. This exercise targets the upper body, including the chest, shoulders, triceps, and core, making it an excellent addition to any fitness routine focused on building strength and stability without the need for heavy weights or equipment. Here's a detailed guide on how to perform Wall Push-Ups, along with the benefits they offer.

Instructions:

1. Begin by standing facing a wall, approximately an arm's length away. Place your palms flat against the wall at shoulder height and shoulder-width apart.
2. Keep your feet planted firmly on the ground, shoulder-width apart. This is your starting position.
3. Engage your core and keep your body in a straight line from your head to your heels.
4. Inhale as you slowly bend your elbows, bringing your chest towards the wall in a controlled movement. Keep your elbows close to your body rather than flaring them out to the sides.
5. Pause briefly when your nose almost touches the wall.

6. Exhale as you push yourself back to the starting position, straightening your arms and focusing on engaging the muscles in your chest and arms.
7. Aim for 10 to 15 repetitions or as many as you can perform with good form. As you build strength, you can increase the number of repetitions.

Benefits:

Wall Push-Ups are an ideal exercise for women over 40 for several reasons. Firstly, they are low impact, reducing the risk of injury and making them suitable for those with joint concerns or beginners to exercise. By strengthening the upper body, they help improve posture, which is crucial for overall health and can decrease the risk of back pain, a common issue as we age.

Additionally, these exercises engage the core muscles, promoting better balance and stability, both of which are essential for daily activities and preventing falls. The Wall Push-Up is also easily modifiable; by adjusting the distance of your feet from the wall, you can control the difficulty of the exercise, making it adaptable to various fitness levels.

Furthermore, consistent practice of Wall Push-Ups can lead to improved muscle tone and endurance in the upper body, contributing to a more toned appearance. For women over 40, maintaining muscle mass is vital for metabolic health, bone density, and overall vitality.

Triceps Push-Up With Side Leg Lift

The Triceps Push-Up with Side Leg Lift is a nuanced exercise that combines upper body strengthening with balance and coordination, making it an ideal addition to a Wall Pilates Workout for women over 40. This exercise targets not just the triceps but also engages the core and lower body, offering a comprehensive workout that can improve overall fitness and functional strength.

Instructions:

1. Start by standing side-on to a wall, with your feet together and the side of your closest hand to the wall extended towards it at chest level.

2. Place your palm flat against the wall, ensuring your arm is straight and your body is at a slight angle to the wall. This will be your starting position.

3. Engage your core and keep your body in a straight line as you bend your elbow, bringing your torso closer to the wall in a push-up motion.

4. As you press back to the starting position, lift your outside leg sideways off the ground, keeping it straight. This adds a balance challenge and engages the abductors on the side of your hip.

5. Lower your leg as you move into your next triceps push-up, ensuring smooth movements and controlled breathing.

6. Aim for a set of 8-12 repetitions on one side before switching to the other, maintaining a focus on form and alignment throughout.

Benefits:

This exercise is particularly beneficial for women over 40 for several reasons:

- Upper Body Strength: It strengthens the triceps, shoulders, and chest, which is crucial for maintaining functional upper body strength and performing daily activities with ease.

- Core Engagement: The necessity to maintain a straight line from head to heels while performing the push-up and leg lift requires significant core strength, thereby improving stability and reducing the risk of back pain.

- Balance and Coordination: The addition of the side leg lift introduces a balance challenge, enhancing proprioception (body awareness) and coordination, which are essential for preventing falls and maintaining mobility.

- Lower Body Activation: Lifting the leg not only works the abductors and glutes but also engages the leg muscles, making this a well-rounded exercise.

- Flexibility: The dynamic nature of the exercise can help improve flexibility in the hips and shoulders, contributing to a greater range of motion.

Wall Arm Circles

Wall Arm Circles are an effective upper body exercise in a Wall Pilates workout, particularly beneficial for women over 40. This exercise focuses on enhancing shoulder mobility, strengthening the upper back, arms, and improving posture, which is vital for maintaining bone health and reducing the risk of injuries as we age.

Instructions:

1. Begin by standing with your back flat against the wall. Your feet should be shoulder-width apart, a few inches away from the wall, to maintain balance.
2. Extend your arms out to the sides at shoulder height, ensuring that your arms, shoulders, and the back of your hands are in contact with the wall.
3. Slowly start making small circles with your arms, keeping them straight and pressed against the wall. Ensure the movement originates from the shoulders.
4. Perform the circles in a clockwise direction for 10 to 15 repetitions, then switch to counterclockwise for an equal number of repetitions.
5. Focus on maintaining a slow and controlled movement, ensuring your arms stay in contact with the wall throughout the exercise.
6. Gradually increase the size of the circles as your shoulder mobility improves, but ensure the range of motion is comfortable and does not cause any pain.

7. To finish, gently lower your arms down by your sides, taking a moment to feel the engagement in your shoulder muscles.

Benefits:

Wall Arm Circles offer numerous benefits for women over 40 engaging in a Wall Pilates workout. Firstly, they enhance shoulder mobility and flexibility, which is crucial for everyday activities and reducing the risk of shoulder injuries. The exercise also strengthens the muscles around the shoulders, upper back, and arms, contributing to a more toned appearance.

Additionally, this exercise promotes better posture by engaging and strengthening the postural muscles. Improved posture contributes to a reduced strain on the spine and can alleviate common issues such as back pain. Performing Wall Arm Circles regularly can also increase blood circulation to the upper body, aiding in muscle recovery and reducing stiffness.

For women over 40, incorporating Wall Arm Circles into their Pilates routine can lead to increased upper body strength, which is essential for bone health. Weight-bearing exercises like this can help combat the onset of osteoporosis, a concern for women as they age. Moreover, the simplicity and accessibility of the exercise make it an excellent addition to any fitness routine, requiring no equipment and minimal space.

Wall T Push-Up

The Wall T Push-Up is an innovative exercise within the Wall Pilates Workout designed for women over 40, aiming to strengthen the upper body without the need for heavy weights or equipment. This exercise is particularly beneficial because it focuses on the shoulders, chest, and upper back, areas that are crucial for maintaining good posture and functional strength as we age. The Wall T Push-Up modifies the traditional floor push-up, making it more accessible and reducing strain on the wrists and shoulders, which can be a concern for many women in this age group.

Instructions for the Wall T Push-Up:

1. Start by standing an arm's length away from a wall, facing it.
2. Extend your arms out to the sides at shoulder height and place your palms flat against the wall, fingers pointing upwards, forming a "T" shape with your body.
3. Keep your feet hip-width apart, ensuring a stable stance.
4. Engage your core and glutes to keep your body in a straight line from head to heels.
5. Inhale as you slowly bend your elbows out to the sides, lowering your chest towards the wall.
6. Exhale as you push back to the starting position, focusing on using your chest and shoulder muscles to move your body.

7. Perform 2-3 sets of 8-12 repetitions, adjusting the number of sets and reps as needed based on your fitness level.

Benefits of the Wall T Push-Up:

The Wall T Push-Up offers numerous benefits, making it an excellent addition to a Wall Pilates Workout for women over 40:

- Strengthens the Upper Body: This exercise targets the chest, shoulders, and upper back muscles, improving overall upper body strength.
- Improves Posture: By strengthening the muscles around the shoulders and upper back, it helps counteract the forward slouching posture that can develop from prolonged sitting or standing.
- Enhances Functional Fitness: Strong shoulders and arms improve daily activities that involve lifting, reaching, or pushing, making tasks easier and reducing the risk of injury.
- Low Impact: Performing push-ups against the wall significantly reduces the strain on the wrists and shoulders, making it a safe alternative for those with joint concerns or limited mobility.
- Adjustable Difficulty: The intensity of the exercise can be easily adjusted by changing the distance of your feet from the wall. Moving your feet further away increases the challenge, while stepping closer reduces it.

- Promotes Bone Health: Weight-bearing exercises like the Wall T Push-Up can help in maintaining bone density, which is particularly important for women over 40, who are at increased risk for osteoporosis.

Lower Body Exercises

Wall Bridge

The "Wall Bridge" is a pivotal exercise in the realm of Wall Pilates, especially designed with women over 40 in mind. This exercise harmoniously blends the principles of Pilates with the structural support of a wall to enhance lower body strength, flexibility, and core stability. The Wall Bridge primarily targets the glutes, hamstrings, lower back, and pelvic muscles, making it an essential component of a comprehensive lower body workout.

Instructions for performing the Wall Bridge are as follows:

1. Begin by lying on your back on a mat, with your legs bent and feet flat on the floor. Move close enough to the wall so that when you extend your legs upward, your feet rest against the wall, hips-width apart.

2. Ensure your arms are by your sides, palms facing down, to provide stability.

3. Press your feet into the wall as you slowly lift your hips towards the ceiling, squeezing your glutes at the top of the movement. Your body should form a straight line from your shoulders to your knees.

4. Hold the bridge position for a few seconds, focusing on tightening your core and glutes.

5. Gently lower your hips back down to the mat in a controlled manner, vertebra by vertebra.

6. Repeat the movement for a set number of repetitions, typically 10-15, depending on your fitness level.

The benefits of incorporating the Wall Bridge into a Wall Pilates workout for women over 40 are multifaceted:

- Enhanced Core Stability: This exercise engages the deep abdominal muscles, improving overall core strength and stability, which is crucial for maintaining balance and preventing falls.

- Lower Back Pain Relief: By strengthening the lower back and improving flexibility, the Wall Bridge can alleviate discomfort and stiffness in the lumbar region, a common issue for many women over 40.

- Improved Posture: Regular practice of this exercise helps correct postural imbalances by strengthening the back and pelvic muscles, encouraging proper alignment.

- Increased Lower Body Strength: Targeting the glutes and hamstrings, the Wall Bridge effectively builds muscle endurance and strength in the lower body, supporting daily movements and physical activities.

- Flexibility and Range of Motion: The controlled movement helps increase the flexibility of the hip flexors and strengthens the pelvic area, enhancing the range of motion.

- Pelvic Floor Health: This exercise also benefits pelvic floor health by engaging and strengthening these muscles, which is especially important for women in their forties and beyond.

Wall Single-Leg Squat

The Wall Single-Leg Squat is an impactful lower body exercise within the Wall Pilates Workout, particularly beneficial for women over 40. This exercise focuses on enhancing strength, stability, and balance by engaging the muscles in a targeted and controlled manner. It's designed to strengthen the quadriceps, hamstrings, glutes, and core muscles, while also challenging balance and coordination, making it a comprehensive workout that addresses many of the physical concerns women face as they age.

Instructions for performing the Wall Single-Leg Squat:

1. Start by standing with your back against a wall, feet hip-width apart. Distance yourself about two feet away from the wall for stability.

2. Engage your core muscles to provide stability and support throughout the exercise.

3. Shift your weight onto your right foot, lifting your left foot off the ground slightly in front of you. Keep your left leg active and straight, with toes pointing forward.

4. Begin to slide down the wall by bending your right knee, keeping your torso straight and ensuring your right knee does not extend past your toes.

5. Lower yourself to a challenging yet manageable depth, aiming for a position where your thigh is parallel to the floor, resembling a seated position.

6. Pause at the bottom of the movement, maintaining balance and control.

7. Pressing through your right heel, straighten your right leg to return to the starting position.

8. Complete the desired number of repetitions on the right leg before switching to the left leg.

Benefits of the Wall Single-Leg Squat for Women Over 40:

1. Strengthens Lower Body Muscles: This exercise targets the quadriceps, hamstrings, and glutes, which are crucial for everyday activities such as walking, climbing stairs, and lifting objects.

2. Improves Balance and Coordination: Performing squats on one leg requires and develops balance and coordination, which can diminish with age, helping to prevent falls and improve overall stability.

3. Enhances Core Stability: The need to maintain an upright posture against the wall engages the core muscles, including the abdominals and lower back, improving posture and reducing the risk of back pain.

4. Increases Joint Health: The controlled movement helps to increase flexibility and range of motion in the knees and hips, contributing to healthier, more lubricated joints.

5. Adaptable to Fitness Levels: By adjusting the depth of the squat and the number of repetitions, this exercise can be modified to match an individual's fitness level, making it accessible for beginners and challenging for those more advanced.

6. Convenient and Accessible: No special equipment is needed besides a wall, making this exercise easy to incorporate into a home workout routine.

7. Supports Weight Management: Like all strength training exercises, Wall Single-Leg Squats help to build muscle mass, which can boost metabolism and aid in weight management.

Wall Squat with Heel Raise

The "Wall Squat with Heel Raise" is a dynamic exercise that enhances the traditional wall squat by incorporating a heel raise to further engage the lower body muscles, making it an excellent addition to a Wall Pilates Workout for women over 40. This exercise targets the quadriceps, hamstrings, calves, and glutes, and also challenges balance and core stability. Here's how to perform the "Wall Squat with Heel Raise" correctly:

- Start by standing with your back against a wall. Place your feet shoulder-width apart and a short distance away from the wall. Your feet should be flat on the ground.
- Slowly slide your back down the wall, bending your knees to lower your body into a squat position. Aim to create a 90-degree angle with your knees, ensuring they are aligned over your ankles, not extending past your toes.
- Press your back, shoulders, and head gently against the wall, engaging your core to maintain stability.
- Once in the squat position, press down through the balls of your feet to lift your heels off the ground, rising onto your toes.
- Hold the heel raise for a moment, then slowly lower your heels back to the floor.
- Press through your feet to slide back up the wall to the starting position.

- Repeat for a set number of repetitions, typically 8-12 for beginners or more as your strength and endurance improve.

Benefits of the Wall Squat with Heel Raise for Women Over 40:

1. Strengthens Lower Body Muscles: This exercise effectively targets and strengthens the quadriceps, hamstrings, calves, and glutes, which are crucial for daily activities and overall mobility.
2. Improves Balance and Stability: By adding the heel raise, this exercise challenges your balance and engages the core, helping to improve your overall stability and posture.
3. Enhances Joint Health: Performing squats against the wall can help in maintaining or improving joint health, particularly in the knees and ankles, by strengthening the muscles around these joints.
4. Increases Bone Density: Weight-bearing exercises like the wall squat with heel raise can help in increasing bone density, which is particularly important for women over 40 as they are at a higher risk of osteoporosis.
5. Boosts Functional Fitness: This exercise mirrors movements you might do in everyday life, such as standing up from a chair or climbing stairs, thereby enhancing your functional fitness and making daily activities easier.
6. Accessible and Safe: Using the wall for support makes this exercise safer and more accessible for individuals who may have balance concerns or are new to strength training, providing a way to build strength without heavy equipment.

7. Flexible and Convenient: It can be done anywhere there is wall space, making it a flexible addition to any fitness routine, especially for those who prefer or need to exercise at home.

Wall Reverse Lunges

Wall Reverse Lunges are a pivotal component of the Wall Pilates Workout, particularly beneficial for women over 40. This exercise seamlessly integrates the principles of Pilates—core stability, balance, and controlled movements—with strength training to target the lower body. By incorporating the wall as a support tool, Wall Reverse Lunges become accessible, offering a safe way to enhance leg strength, improve balance, and increase hip flexibility, which are crucial for maintaining an active lifestyle and preventing injuries as we age.

Instructions:

1. Stand facing away from the wall, with your feet hip-width apart. Place your hands on your hips for added balance.
2. Step forward slightly with one foot to create enough space for the movement.
3. Lean your back gently against the wall for support. This helps maintain an upright posture throughout the exercise.
4. Shift your weight to your front foot.
5. Slowly step backward with your other foot, lowering your body until the back knee gently taps or comes close to the ground. Ensure your front knee is aligned over your ankle and does not extend past your toes.
6. Press through the heel of your front foot to return to the starting position.

7. Repeat the movement for a set number of repetitions before switching legs.

The benefits of Wall Reverse Lunges for women over 40 are manifold. Firstly, they strengthen the major muscles of the legs, including the quadriceps, hamstrings, and glutes, which are essential for everyday activities like climbing stairs, lifting objects, and even maintaining a standing posture. Strengthening these muscles also contributes to a reduction in the risk of falls, a common concern as we age.

Additionally, by engaging the core muscles to maintain stability during the exercise, Wall Reverse Lunges also help to improve core strength and posture. A strong core is vital for preventing lower back pain, a common ailment that can be exacerbated by weak abdominal and back muscles.

Wall Reverse Lunges also promote flexibility in the hip flexors, muscles that can become tight due to prolonged periods of sitting. This tightness can lead to lower back discomfort and reduced mobility. By regularly performing lunges, flexibility can be improved, leading to better movement patterns and reduced discomfort.

Another key benefit is the enhancement of balance. As balance can decline with age, incorporating exercises that challenge and improve this aspect of fitness is crucial. The wall provides a support mechanism, allowing for the focus to be on the quality of movement rather than on maintaining balance, making the exercise more accessible for those who may struggle with balance.

Lastly, Wall Reverse Lunges can be easily modified to increase or decrease intensity, making them suitable for a range of fitness levels. For those seeking more of a challenge, adding weights or increasing the number of repetitions can provide further strength benefits.

Single-Leg Bridge With Abduction

The Single-Leg Bridge With Abduction is a pivotal exercise in the realm of Wall Pilates, especially curated for women over 40. This exercise not only targets the lower body, focusing on the glutes, hamstrings, and inner thighs, but also incorporates core stabilization and balance, making it an invaluable addition to any workout regimen for enhancing overall strength and mobility.

To perform the Single-Leg Bridge With Abduction effectively, one should follow these structured steps:

1. Begin by lying on your back with your feet flat against the wall, knees bent, and arms resting by your sides for stability.

2. Press one foot firmly into the wall while extending the other leg straight out in alignment with the bent knee. This is your starting position.

3. Engage your core and lift your hips towards the ceiling, pressing the foot on the wall to elevate your body into a bridge position. Ensure your spine remains neutral and your hips are level.

4. Once stabilized in the bridge, slowly abduct the extended leg by moving it away from the midline of your body, then bring it back to the center. Keep your movements controlled and deliberate.

5. Lower your hips back to the floor to return to the starting position.
6. Repeat the sequence for a set number of repetitions before switching legs.

The benefits of incorporating the Single-Leg Bridge With Abduction into a Wall Pilates Workout for women over 40 are multifaceted. Firstly, it strengthens the gluteal muscles and hamstrings, which are crucial for lower back support, improved posture, and injury prevention. Moreover, the abduction movement activates the inner and outer thighs, enhancing leg tonality and promoting hip stability.

This exercise also emphasizes core engagement throughout the movement, which aids in developing a stronger, more supportive core. A robust core is essential for maintaining balance, improving overall movement efficiency, and reducing the risk of falls. Additionally, the Single-Leg Bridge With Abduction can help improve flexibility in the hip flexors, a common area of tightness for many, especially those who spend long periods sitting.

For women over 40, maintaining muscle mass and bone density is paramount, and resistance exercises like this play a key role in achieving such health objectives. By utilizing the resistance provided by the wall, this exercise also offers a safe way to increase intensity without the need for additional weights, making it accessible for those with varying levels of fitness.

Wall Glute Bridge March

The Wall Glute Bridge March is a versatile exercise that combines the stability and resistance of a wall with the benefits of traditional Pilates, making it particularly beneficial for women over 40. This exercise focuses on strengthening the lower body, with a special emphasis on the glutes, hamstrings, and core muscles. It also helps improve balance and stability, which are crucial for maintaining an active lifestyle and preventing falls as we age.

To perform the Wall Glute Bridge March, follow these instructions:

1. Begin by lying on your back with your feet flat against the wall. Your legs should be bent at a 90-degree angle, and your feet should be hip-width apart.
2. Press your arms and palms down into the floor alongside your body for stability.
3. Engage your core and lift your hips towards the ceiling, pressing your feet into the wall to create a straight line from your shoulders to your knees. This is your starting position.
4. From this bridge position, slowly lift one foot off the wall, bringing your knee towards your chest, while keeping your hips elevated and stable.
5. Lower your foot back to the wall and repeat with the other leg, continuing to alternate legs as if marching on the spot.

6. Focus on keeping your pelvis stable and your movements controlled. Avoid letting your hips sag or twist.

7. Perform 10-15 marches on each leg, maintaining the lifted hip position throughout.

The benefits of incorporating the Wall Glute Bridge March into your Pilates routine are numerous, especially for women over 40:

- Strengthens the Glutes and Hamstrings: This exercise targets the glutes and hamstrings, which are key to lower body strength, stability, and injury prevention.

- Core Activation: Maintaining the bridge position requires significant core engagement, which strengthens the abdominal muscles and supports spinal health.

- Improves Balance and Stability: The alternating leg movements challenge your balance, improving stability and coordination.

- Enhances Flexibility: The movement helps increase flexibility in the hip flexors, which is beneficial for those who spend a lot of time sitting.

- Low Impact: This exercise is gentle on the joints, making it ideal for those who need or prefer low-impact workouts.

- Adaptable: The difficulty level can be easily adjusted by changing the height of the feet on the wall or the tempo of the marches, making it suitable for various fitness levels.

Leg and Glute Exercises

Wall Leg Lifts

Wall leg lifts are a pivotal component of the Wall Pilates Workout designed for women over 40, targeting the strengthening and toning of the legs and glutes. This exercise utilizes the stability and resistance provided by the wall to enhance the effectiveness of the movement, ensuring a safe and supportive environment for those who may be concerned about balance and joint stress.

To perform wall leg lifts correctly:

1. Begin by standing side-on to the wall, your body straight and one hand resting on the wall for balance.
2. Keep your feet hip-width apart, and your gaze forward, ensuring your posture is upright and engaged.
3. Slowly lift the leg closest to the wall upwards, keeping it straight, to a comfortable height. The goal is to feel a stretch in the inner thigh of the lifting leg and engagement in the glutes.
4. Hold the lifted position for a moment, then slowly lower your leg back down, maintaining control and not allowing your foot to crash back to the floor.
5. Perform the desired number of repetitions on one leg before switching to the other side, ensuring both legs receive equal attention.

The benefits of incorporating wall leg lifts into a Pilates regimen for women over 40 are numerous. Firstly, this exercise promotes leg strength, vital for maintaining mobility and reducing the risk of falls as we age. Secondly, it aids in toning the gluteal muscles, which is essential for posture and back support. Thirdly, wall leg lifts can enhance flexibility in the hips and improve circulation in the lower limbs, contributing to overall leg health.

Moreover, the wall provides a form of resistance that can be adjusted according to one's strength and flexibility levels, making wall leg lifts a highly adaptable exercise. It allows for gradual progression, which is crucial for building strength safely and effectively without the risk of injury. Additionally, the support from the wall ensures that the exercise is low-impact, making it suitable for those with joint concerns or who are new to fitness routines.

Incorporating wall leg lifts into a regular Pilates workout offers a pathway to improved balance and coordination. The necessity to maintain an upright posture while performing the lifts encourages core engagement, which is beneficial for balance. This core activation, combined with the strengthening of the legs and glutes, contributes significantly to enhanced coordination and stability, both of which are crucial for daily activities.

Lastly, the simplicity of wall leg lifts means they can easily be integrated into any workout routine, requiring no special equipment other than a wall. This makes them an accessible exercise option for women over 40 looking to incorporate effective leg and glute exercises into their fitness routines, whether at home or in a studio setting.

Through consistent practice, wall leg lifts can significantly contribute to a stronger, more toned lower body, improved posture, and enhanced balance and coordination, making them a valuable addition to a Wall Pilates Workout for women over 40.

Wall Side Leg Lifts

Wall Side Leg Lifts are a pivotal component of a Wall Pilates Workout, especially designed for women over 40, focusing on strengthening the legs and glutes while improving balance and stability. This exercise, when performed correctly, can offer a multitude of benefits, making it a must-add to any fitness regimen for those looking to enhance their physical well-being in midlife and beyond.

To execute Wall Side Leg Lifts effectively, follow these steps:

1. Start by standing parallel to the wall, with your body's side facing the wall. Ensure that you're close enough so that your fingertips can lightly touch the wall for balance.
2. Place your feet together, standing tall with your back straight and your core engaged.
3. Slowly lift the leg that is furthest from the wall upwards, keeping it straight. The goal is to raise it as high as comfortably possible without compromising form.
4. Pause briefly at the top of the lift to maximize the engagement of the glute muscles.
5. Lower the leg back down with control, maintaining the alignment and not allowing your foot to crash back to the starting position.

6. Repeat the movement for the desired number of repetitions before switching sides and performing the exercise with the other leg.

The benefits of incorporating Wall Side Leg Lifts into a Wall Pilates workout for women over 40 are extensive:
- Strengthens the Lower Body: This exercise targets the glutes, hamstrings, and abductors, contributing to stronger, more toned legs.

- Improves Balance and Stability: As you age, maintaining balance becomes crucial. Wall Side Leg Lifts help improve your balance, reducing the risk of falls.

- Enhances Core Engagement: Although the focus is on the legs and glutes, maintaining your balance and posture during this exercise also engages your core, contributing to improved core strength and stability.

- Increases Flexibility: Regularly performing this exercise can help increase the range of motion in your hips and legs.

- Accessible and Safe: For women over 40, safety during exercise is paramount. The wall serves as a support, making this exercise less likely to cause injury while still offering significant fitness benefits.

- Adaptable to Fitness Levels: You can easily adjust the intensity of this exercise by modifying the height of the leg lift according to your fitness level and flexibility.

Wall Single Leg Lifts

Wall Single Leg Lifts are a pivotal exercise within the Wall Pilates Workout, specifically tailored for women over 40. This exercise focuses on strengthening the legs and glutes, areas that often require attention as the body matures. The beauty of Wall Single Leg Lifts lies in their simplicity and effectiveness, providing a low-impact option that significantly impacts muscle toning and stability enhancement.

To perform Wall Single Leg Lifts correctly, follow these steps:

1. Stand with your side to the wall, placing one hand on the wall for support.
2. Keep your standing leg slightly bent to engage the muscles and ensure stability.
3. Slowly lift the leg closest to the wall upwards, keeping it straight. Your body should form a slight "T" shape.
4. Hold the lift for a moment at the top of the movement, ensuring you feel the engagement in your glutes and the side of your thigh.
5. Lower the leg back down with control, aiming for a smooth, steady motion.
6. Repeat the exercise for the desired number of repetitions before switching sides to ensure both legs are worked evenly.

The benefits of incorporating Wall Single Leg Lifts into a Pilates regimen for women over 40 are manifold. Firstly, this exercise strengthens the quadriceps, hamstrings, and gluteal muscles, which is crucial for maintaining leg strength and overall mobility. Strengthening these muscle groups can help in reducing the risk of injuries and improving balance, both of which become increasingly important with age.

Additionally, Wall Single Leg Lifts can enhance core stability. Although the primary focus is on the legs and glutes, maintaining balance and the correct posture during the exercise engages the core muscles, including the abdominals and lower back. This inadvertent engagement helps in toning the core and improving posture, contributing to a reduced risk of lower back pain, a common ailment among adults over 40.

Another significant benefit is the promotion of muscular symmetry and balance. By isolating each leg during the exercise, Wall Single Leg Lifts ensure that both the dominant and non-dominant sides of the body are equally strengthened. This balance is vital for functional movements and can help in correcting muscular imbalances, thereby enhancing overall physical performance.

Furthermore, Wall Single Leg Lifts are easily modifiable to suit various fitness levels. For those seeking a greater challenge, ankle weights can be added, or the range of motion can be increased.

Conversely, for beginners or those with balance issues, the lift height can be adjusted to a more manageable level.

Lastly, the low-impact nature of Wall Single Leg Lifts makes them an ideal exercise for women over 40, particularly those with joint concerns or who are new to exercise. By supporting some of the body's weight against the wall, the exercise reduces the strain on the knees and hips, making it a safe and effective way to build strength.

Wall Mountain Climbers

Wall Mountain Climbers, tailored for the Wall Pilates Workout for Women Over 40, offers a unique twist on the traditional floor-based mountain climbers. This variation brings a focus on engaging and strengthening the legs and glutes, crucial for maintaining muscle tone, balance, and stability as we age. The vertical element of the wall adds an interesting challenge, promoting core engagement and enhancing overall body coordination in a low-impact format suitable for those concerned about joint health.

Instructions:

1. Start by facing the wall, standing arms' length away. Place your hands against the wall at shoulder height and shoulder-width apart.
2. Lean into the wall, forming a strong, straight line with your body, similar to the starting position of a push-up against the wall.
3. Begin by lifting your right knee towards your chest, keeping the toes pointed and engaging your core muscles to maintain stability.
4. Return the right leg to the starting position and then switch, lifting the left knee towards the chest. The movement mimics running in place against the wall.
5. Continue alternating legs at a controlled pace, focusing on form and the engagement of the core, legs, and glutes.

Benefits:

- Enhanced Core Stability: This exercise requires significant core engagement to maintain balance and posture against the wall, leading to improved core strength and stability.

- Lower Body Strength: The lifting and lowering action of the legs, against gravity and with the added resistance of the wall, intensify the workout for the quadriceps, hamstrings, and glutes.

- Cardiovascular Health: The dynamic movement of switching legs quickly can increase heart rate, offering cardiovascular benefits similar to those of low-impact aerobic activities.

- Improved Balance and Coordination: Performing mountain climbers against a wall requires and develops a good sense of balance and body coordination, which are vital for functional movements in daily activities.

- Joint-Friendly: For women over 40, especially those with knee or hip concerns, wall mountain climbers provide a safer alternative to high-impact exercises, reducing the strain on joints while still offering an effective workout.

Kneeling Side Leg Lift

The Kneeling Side Leg Lift is a valuable exercise within the Wall Pilates Workout, especially tailored for women over 40. This exercise focuses on strengthening the legs and glutes, areas that are crucial for maintaining overall balance, stability, and a strong foundation. It also targets the core muscles, promoting better posture and reducing the risk of injuries by enhancing muscular coordination and flexibility.

Instructions for performing the Kneeling Side Leg Lift:

1. Begin by kneeling on a mat with your left side near the wall, keeping your body aligned straight from your head to your knees.
2. Place your left hand on the floor directly under your shoulder for support, and rest your right hand on the wall for balance.
3. Extend your right leg out to the side, keeping it straight and in line with your body. Your left knee should remain on the mat, and your right foot should be flexed.
4. Slowly lift your right leg upwards towards the wall without shifting your hips or leaning towards the wall. Ensure the movement is controlled and originates from the glutes and hip abductors.
5. Hold the lifted position briefly at the top of the movement, then slowly lower the leg back down to the

starting position, without letting your foot touch the ground completely.

6. Repeat the lift for the desired number of repetitions before switching to the other side.

Benefits of the Kneeling Side Leg Lift:

- Strengthens the gluteus medius and minimus, crucial muscles for hip stability and movement.
- Enhances core stability as the exercise requires balance and coordination, engaging the abdominal muscles to maintain posture.
- Improves flexibility and range of motion in the hips, contributing to smoother, more efficient movements in daily activities.
- Supports better posture by strengthening the muscles along the side of the body, helping to prevent the natural tendency towards slouching.
- Reduces the risk of lower back pain by balancing the muscular strength around the pelvis, providing better support for the lower spine.
- Can aid in the prevention of knee injuries by ensuring the muscles surrounding the hips are strong and capable of supporting the joints during various activities.
- Offers a low-impact option for leg and glute strengthening, making it ideal for women over 40 who may be looking for effective exercises that do not strain the joints.

Wall Toe Taps

Wall Toe Taps as part of a Wall Pilates Workout are a fantastic exercise for women over 40 looking to strengthen their lower body, particularly targeting the legs and glutes. This exercise is not only beneficial for toning muscles but also for improving balance and stability, which are crucial for overall mobility and injury prevention as we age. Here's a closer look at how to perform Wall Toe Taps and the benefits they offer.

Instructions for Wall Toe Taps:

1. Begin by standing with your back against a wall, feet hip-width apart, and arms by your sides. Ensure your entire back is flat against the wall for support.
2. Engage your core muscles to stabilize your spine and pelvis throughout the exercise.
3. Slowly lift one foot off the ground, bending the knee to bring the thigh parallel to the floor, creating a 90-degree angle at the knee.
4. Gently tap the toes of the lifted foot to the ground, then raise the foot back to the starting position.
5. Repeat this motion for a set number of repetitions before switching legs.
6. Keep the movement controlled and focused, paying particular attention to maintaining balance and stability with your back against the wall.

7. Breathe evenly throughout the exercise, exhaling as you lift your leg, and inhaling as you lower it.

Benefits of Wall Toe Taps:

1. Muscle Strengthening and Toning: Wall Toe Taps primarily target the quadriceps, hamstrings, and gluteal muscles. Regularly performing this exercise can help tone and strengthen these areas, leading to improved muscle definition and strength.

2. Improved Balance and Stability: By performing this exercise with your back against the wall, you challenge your balance and stability. Over time, this can lead to better posture and reduced risk of falls, which is particularly beneficial for women over 40.

3. Core Engagement: Although the focus is on the legs and glutes, Wall Toe Taps require significant core engagement to maintain stability and posture. This can lead to a stronger core, which is essential for overall body strength and injury prevention.

4. Low Impact: For women over 40, especially those with joint concerns or who are new to exercise, Wall Toe Taps offer a low-impact option that minimizes stress on the knees and ankles.

5. Accessibility: This exercise doesn't require any special equipment and can be performed anywhere there's a wall, making it an excellent option for home workouts or when traveling.

6. Flexibility Improvement: Regularly performing Wall Toe Taps can help improve the flexibility of the hip flexors and leg muscles, contributing to a greater range of motion and reducing the risk of muscle strains.

7. Enhanced Coordination: As a unilateral exercise that requires balancing on one leg at a time, Wall Toe Taps can help improve coordination and proprioception, which are important for daily activities and other forms of exercise.

Flexibility and Mobility Exercises

Wall Hip Stretch

The Wall Hip Stretch is a pivotal component of a Wall Pilates Workout, especially designed for women over 40 who are looking to enhance their flexibility and mobility. As we age, maintaining hip flexibility is crucial for performing daily activities with ease, reducing lower back pain, and improving overall movement quality. This exercise specifically targets the muscles around the hip joint, including the hip flexors, glutes, and inner thigh muscles, offering a gentle yet effective stretch that can be easily incorporated into a Pilates routine.

To perform the Wall Hip Stretch, follow these steps:

1. Begin by standing facing the wall, approximately an arm's length away. Place your hands on the wall at shoulder height for stability.
2. Step back with one foot, keeping it straight, and press the heel firmly into the ground. The other foot remains in front, with the knee slightly bent.
3. Lean forward into the wall, keeping your back straight, and push your hips back. You should feel a stretch in the hip of the leg that is extended behind you.

4. Hold this position for 20-30 seconds, breathing deeply to allow your muscles to relax and stretch further.

5. Gently release the stretch and switch legs, repeating the stretch on the other side.

6. For a deeper stretch, you can adjust the distance of your back foot from the wall or increase the bend in your front knee, always ensuring you maintain good posture and do not strain your muscles.

The benefits of incorporating the Wall Hip Stretch into a Wall Pilates Workout for women over 40 are manifold. Firstly, it helps to counteract the stiffness and reduced mobility that can come with age, particularly around the hip area which is prone to tightness from prolonged sitting or standing. This stretch aids in improving the range of motion, making daily movements smoother and more fluid.

Furthermore, by enhancing hip flexibility, this stretch can also contribute to better posture. Tight hip flexors can pull on the lower back, leading to discomfort and slouching. Regularly performing the Wall Hip Stretch can alleviate this tension, promoting a more upright and aligned posture.

Additionally, the Wall Hip Stretch is beneficial for preventing injuries. Flexible hips can absorb shock and stress more effectively, reducing the risk of strains and sprains during physical activity. For women over 40, who may be concerned about injury, this is particularly important.

This exercise also plays a role in balancing muscle strength and flexibility across the body. By ensuring the hips are adequately stretched, it can prevent muscle imbalances that might lead to compensatory movements and potential discomfort or injury elsewhere in the body.

Lastly, the Wall Hip Stretch offers a moment of mindfulness and relaxation. Focusing on deep, controlled breathing during the stretch can have a calming effect, reducing stress and enhancing the mind-body connection that is central to Pilates practice.

Wall Shoulder Stretch

The Wall Shoulder Stretch is an essential part of a Wall Pilates Workout, especially designed for women over 40, focusing on improving flexibility and mobility in the shoulder region. As we age, maintaining shoulder mobility becomes crucial for performing daily activities and reducing the risk of injuries. This stretch is particularly beneficial because it targets the muscles around the shoulders and upper back, areas that often become tight due to poor posture or prolonged periods of sitting.

To perform the Wall Shoulder Stretch, follow these instructions:

1. Stand facing a wall, approximately an arm's length away.
2. Extend your right arm and place your palm against the wall at shoulder height, fingers pointing towards the ceiling.
3. Keeping your arm straight, slowly turn your body away from the wall until you feel a gentle stretch across the front of your shoulder and chest.
4. Hold this position for 15 to 30 seconds, breathing deeply to allow your muscles to relax into the stretch.
5. Gently release and repeat the stretch with your left arm.
6. For a deeper stretch, move your hand higher up the wall or step further away from the wall before turning your body.

The benefits:

- Improved Flexibility: Regularly performing this stretch can help increase the range of motion in your shoulders, making it easier to reach overhead and perform various Pilates movements.

- Reduced Tension and Pain: This stretch helps alleviate tension in the shoulders and upper back, which can reduce discomfort and the risk of strain injuries, particularly beneficial for women over 40 who may experience increased stiffness.

- Enhanced Posture: By stretching the chest and shoulder muscles, this exercise encourages better posture. Over time, this can help counteract the forward shoulder slump that often develops from sitting at a desk or using a smartphone.

- Increased Blood Flow: Stretching the shoulder area increases blood circulation to the muscles, promoting healing and reducing recovery time between workouts.

- Supports Daily Activities: Improved shoulder mobility makes it easier to perform everyday tasks, such as lifting objects or reaching behind, contributing to a better quality of life.

Wall Calf Stretch

The Wall Calf Stretch is a pivotal component of the flexibility and mobility exercises segment in a Wall Pilates Workout, especially tailored for women over 40. This specific stretch is integral for maintaining lower leg health, improving flexibility in the calf muscles, and enhancing overall mobility, which can significantly impact daily activities and the effectiveness of the Pilates practice.

To perform the Wall Calf Stretch, one should follow these organized instructions:

1. Begin by facing a wall, standing about an arm's length away.
2. Extend your arms and place your palms flat against the wall at shoulder height.
3. Step one foot back, keeping it straight, and press the heel firmly into the ground.
4. The other foot should remain in front, with the knee bent.
5. Keep both heels on the ground and press your hips forward towards the wall to deepen the stretch in the calf of the back leg.
6. Hold this position for 20 to 30 seconds, feeling a gentle stretch in the calf muscle.
7. Switch legs and repeat the stretch to ensure both calves are equally worked.

The benefits of integrating the Wall Calf Stretch into a Pilates workout for women over 40 are numerous. Firstly, it helps to prevent injuries that can occur from the stiffening of muscles as one ages. By regularly performing this stretch, the risk of calf strains or tears can be significantly reduced, promoting a safer exercise experience. Additionally, enhanced calf flexibility contributes to a better range of motion in the ankles, which can improve balance and stability—a crucial factor for preventing falls.

Furthermore, this stretch aids in improving circulation in the lower legs, which is beneficial for women experiencing swelling or varicose veins, common issues as the body ages. Improved circulation can also lead to better performance during Pilates exercises and other physical activities by efficiently delivering oxygen to the muscles and removing waste products.

Incorporating the Wall Calf Stretch into a Wall Pilates routine can also alleviate symptoms of plantar fasciitis, a condition that tends to affect individuals over 40. By stretching the calf muscles, tension on the plantar fascia is reduced, providing relief from foot pain associated with this condition.

Moreover, this stretch can enhance proprioception, or the awareness of body position and movement, which is vital for executing Pilates exercises with precision and control. Improved proprioception not only contributes to the effectiveness of the workout but also reduces the likelihood of injury.

Lastly, the Wall Calf Stretch, by promoting flexibility and mobility, can have a positive impact on posture. Tight calf muscles can lead to alterations in the way one walks, which, in turn, can affect posture and lead to back or hip pain. Regularly performing this stretch can help maintain a natural gait and support overall postural alignment.

Wall Chest Opener Stretch

The Wall Chest Opener Stretch is a vital component of the flexibility and mobility exercises within a Wall Pilates Workout, particularly beneficial for women over 40. This stretch is designed to counteract the forward-leaning posture that often develops from daily activities like computer work, driving, or any task that encourages a forward hunch. The Wall Chest Opener targets the chest, shoulders, and biceps, promoting better posture and reducing tension in the upper body.

Instructions for the Wall Chest Opener Stretch include:

- Stand facing sideways next to a wall with your feet hip-width apart.
- Raise the arm closest to the wall to shoulder height, and press your palm against the wall. Fingers should be pointed away from your body.
- Keeping your palm firmly on the wall, slowly rotate your body away from the wall until you feel a stretch across your chest and the front of your shoulder.
- Hold this position, ensuring your arm remains parallel to the floor, and maintain the stretch for 20 to 30 seconds.
- Gently release the stretch by rotating your body back to the starting position.

o Repeat on the other side to ensure balanced flexibility.

- The benefits of incorporating the Wall Chest Opener Stretch into your Wall Pilates routine are manifold, especially for women over 40:
- Improves Posture: This stretch helps realign the shoulders, reducing the rounded forward posture and encouraging a more upright stance.
- Increases Flexibility: Regularly performing this stretch increases flexibility in the chest and shoulders, areas that can become tight from daily activities or lack of movement.
- Enhances Breathing: Opening up the chest allows for deeper, more efficient breathing by expanding the ribcage, which can improve oxygen flow to the muscles and brain.
- Reduces Pain: It can alleviate tension and pain in the neck, shoulders, and upper back by stretching and lengthening the pectoral muscles.
- Prepares for Exercise: This stretch is an excellent preparatory movement for more intensive Pilates exercises, warming up the muscles and joints for a safer and more effective workout.
- Promotes Circulation: Stretching the chest area helps improve blood circulation, which can aid in muscle recovery and reduce soreness after workouts.

Wall Spine Stretch

The Wall Spine Stretch is an invaluable component of a Wall Pilates Workout, especially tailored for women over 40. This exercise focuses on enhancing spinal flexibility and mobility, crucial aspects for maintaining a healthy posture and reducing the risk of back pain, which can become more prevalent with age. The Wall Spine Stretch involves a series of movements that allow the spine to extend and flex while using the wall for support and alignment.

To perform the Wall Spine Stretch, follow these steps:

1. Start by standing with your back against the wall, feet hip-width apart and a slight distance away from the wall. Ensure your entire spine is aligned with the wall.
2. Slowly slide your hands up the wall above your head, stretching your body upwards while keeping your abdominal muscles gently engaged.
3. Begin to peel your spine off the wall, starting from the neck, upper back, and moving downwards, bending forward at the waist as far as comfortable, reaching towards your toes. Keep your hands in contact with the wall for support.
4. Hold the forward bend position briefly to allow your spine to stretch fully.

5. Gently return to the starting position by rolling your spine back against the wall, vertebra by vertebra, until you're standing straight again.

6. Throughout the exercise, focus on smooth, controlled movements to maximize the stretch along your spine.

The benefits of incorporating the Wall Spine Stretch into a Pilates workout regimen for women over 40 are manifold. Firstly, it promotes spinal health by encouraging flexibility in the vertebrae, which can help in alleviating stiffness and discomfort often associated with aging and sedentary lifestyles. Regularly performing this stretch can lead to improved posture, as it strengthens the muscles around the spine, supporting proper alignment.

Additionally, the Wall Spine Stretch enhances overall mobility, making everyday movements easier and reducing the risk of injury. This is particularly important for women over 40, who may be experiencing the beginnings of joint degeneration or osteoporosis. By improving spinal mobility, this exercise helps in maintaining a range of motion, which is essential for a healthy and active lifestyle.

Moreover, the controlled movement and focus on alignment during the Wall Spine Stretch encourage mindfulness and body awareness. This mental engagement with the exercise can have calming effects, reducing stress and enhancing mental clarity. It also fosters a connection between mind and body, a fundamental principle of Pilates, enhancing the overall effectiveness of the workout.

Wall Hamstring Stretch

The Wall Hamstring Stretch is a pivotal component of the Flexibility and Mobility section in a Wall Pilates Workout, particularly beneficial for women over 40. This demographic often faces increased risks of muscle tightness and reduced flexibility due to changes in muscle elasticity and decreased physical activity levels. The Wall Hamstring Stretch directly addresses these concerns by targeting the muscles at the back of the thigh, crucial for daily movements like walking, bending, and squatting.

To perform the Wall Hamstring Stretch, follow these steps:

1. Begin by lying on the floor on your back, close to a wall. Position your buttocks as close to the wall base as possible.
2. Extend your legs upward, resting your heels against the wall. The closer your hips are to the wall, the deeper the stretch.
3. Keep one leg against the wall while slowly lowering the other leg down, bending it at the knee, until a stretch is felt in the hamstring of the extended leg.
4. Hold this position, ensuring your back and tailbone are flat against the floor to maintain the integrity of the stretch.
5. Focus on deep, steady breaths, allowing the hamstring to relax and lengthen with each exhale.
6. After holding for a desired time, usually between 15 to 30 seconds, switch legs and repeat the stretch.

The benefits of incorporating the Wall Hamstring Stretch into your Pilates routine are manifold. Firstly, it enhances flexibility in the hamstrings, which is essential for maintaining an optimal range of motion in the hips and lower back. This can lead to improved posture and reduced discomfort in daily activities.

Secondly, it promotes circulation to the lower body, which is beneficial for muscle recovery and health. Improved blood flow ensures that muscle tissues receive a healthy supply of oxygen and nutrients, aiding in recovery and function.

Furthermore, this stretch can mitigate the risk of back pain, a common ailment among women over 40. Tight hamstrings can contribute to lower back strain by pulling on the pelvis and affecting spinal alignment. Regularly stretching these muscles helps reduce this risk, contributing to a healthier back and more comfortable movement patterns.

Additionally, the Wall Hamstring Stretch can enhance overall mobility, making it easier to engage in physical activities and maintain an active lifestyle. It can serve as a foundation for more dynamic Pilates movements, ensuring that exercises are performed safely and effectively.

Lastly, focusing on flexibility and mobility exercises like the Wall Hamstring Stretch can have a calming effect, reducing stress and promoting relaxation. The focused, gentle nature of the stretch encourages mindfulness and can help in developing a deeper connection between mind and body.

Wall Quad Stretch

The Wall Quad Stretch is a pivotal element in the flexibility and mobility segment of a Wall Pilates Workout, particularly beneficial for women over 40. This exercise focuses on stretching the quadriceps, the muscle group at the front of the thigh, which is crucial for knee health, proper posture, and ease in daily movements such as walking, sitting, and climbing stairs. For women over 40, maintaining flexibility in the quadriceps can help counteract the stiffness and loss of mobility that can come with age, ensuring a more active and injury-free lifestyle.

To perform the Wall Quad Stretch:

1. Stand facing away from the wall, approximately an arm's length distance.
2. Bend your right knee and bring your heel towards your buttocks.
3. Reach back with your right hand and grab your right ankle. If you cannot reach your ankle comfortably, a towel or resistance band looped around the ankle can be used as an extension of your hand.
4. Gently pull your right heel closer to your body, ensuring your knee is pointing straight down towards the floor, not splaying out to the side.
5. Place your left hand on the wall for balance and support.

6. Keep your standing leg slightly bent to avoid locking the knee, and press your hips forward slightly to enhance the stretch in the front of the thigh.

7. Hold the stretch for 20 to 30 seconds, breathing deeply and steadily, then gently release and switch legs.

The benefits of incorporating the Wall Quad Stretch into a Pilates workout regimen for women over 40 are numerous. Firstly, it enhances flexibility in the quadriceps, which can help improve overall leg mobility and reduce the risk of injury from daily activities. Stretching the quads can also alleviate tightness and discomfort in the knee and hip areas, common concerns for women in this age group.

Furthermore, regular performance of the Wall Quad Stretch can aid in correcting posture. Tight quadriceps are often a contributing factor to anterior pelvic tilt, a common postural issue that can lead to lower back pain. By lengthening and loosening the quads, this stretch helps to promote a more neutral pelvic position, contributing to better posture and reduced back discomfort.

In addition to its physical benefits, this stretch, like many Pilates exercises, encourages mindfulness and body awareness. The focused breathing and attention to the stretch's sensation foster a deeper connection between mind and body, enhancing the overall Pilates practice's calming and centering effects.

Lastly, the Wall Quad Stretch is easily modifiable. Women over 40 with varying fitness levels and flexibility can adjust the intensity of the stretch to suit their comfort levels, making it a versatile and inclusive component of any Wall Pilates workout. This adaptability ensures that as flexibility improves, the stretch can be deepened progressively, offering continued benefits and challenges over time.

Special Focus Exercises

Wall Knee Tucks

Wall Knee Tucks within a Wall Pilates Workout specifically designed for women over 40 offer a unique blend of core strengthening, balance improvement, and flexibility enhancement. This exercise targets the abdominal muscles, hips, and lower back, making it a versatile component of a Pilates routine that focuses on areas women over 40 often wish to strengthen and tone.

To perform Wall Knee Tucks correctly, follow these instructions:

1. Start by facing away from the wall, in a plank position, with your feet placed against the wall. Your hands should be directly under your shoulders on the floor, and your body should form a straight line from your head to your heels.
2. Engage your core muscles to stabilize your body.
3. Gently draw one knee towards your chest, using the wall to support the movement of your foot. Keep your back straight and your hips level.
4. Return your foot to the starting position against the wall.
5. Repeat the movement with the other leg.
6. Alternate legs for the desired number of repetitions, ensuring smooth, controlled movements throughout.

The benefits of incorporating Wall Knee Tucks into a Wall Pilates workout are numerous, especially for women over 40. Firstly, this exercise significantly strengthens the core muscles, including the abdominals, lower back, and obliques. A strong core is essential not only for a toned appearance but also for improving posture, reducing back pain, and enhancing balance, which is crucial as balance can start to deteriorate with age.

Additionally, Wall Knee Tucks help to improve hip mobility and flexibility. As the knees are drawn in towards the chest, the hip flexors are actively engaged, which can help to counteract the stiffness and tightness that often come with age, particularly for those who spend a lot of time sitting.

This exercise also has a low impact on the joints, making it an excellent option for those who may have joint concerns or are looking for a workout that is effective yet gentle on the body. Since it's performed against the wall, it allows for more control over the movement, reducing the risk of strain or injury.

Moreover, Wall Knee Tucks encourage concentration and body awareness. Performing the exercise requires focus on maintaining proper form and alignment, which in turn enhances the mind-body connection—a key principle of Pilates.

Finally, this exercise is versatile and easily modified to suit different fitness levels. Beginners can start with fewer repetitions or reduce the range of motion, while more advanced individuals can increase the number of repetitions or add a pause at the knee-to-chest position to intensify the workout.

Wall Oblique Twist

The Wall Oblique Twist is a pivotal exercise in the Wall Pilates Workout for Women Over 40, targeting the core muscles with a special focus on the obliques. This exercise enhances rotational strength, stability, and flexibility, which are essential for daily activities and overall physical health. The obliques play a crucial role in supporting the spine, improving posture, and facilitating efficient movement patterns, making the Wall Oblique Twist a valuable addition to any fitness regimen for women in this age group.

To perform the Wall Oblique Twist effectively, follow these instructions:

1. Stand with your side facing the wall, approximately an arm's length away. Feet should be hip-width apart, ensuring a stable stance.

2. Extend your arms in front of you, keeping them parallel to the ground. The hand closest to the wall should touch the wall lightly.

3. Engage your core muscles to maintain a straight and strong posture throughout the exercise.

4. Rotate your torso towards the wall, leading with the hand touching the wall while keeping your hips facing forward. This movement should be controlled and originate from the waist, emphasizing the twist on the obliques.

5. Return to the starting position, then repeat the twist multiple times before switching sides to ensure balanced strengthening of both oblique muscles.

The benefits:

- Strengthen and tone the oblique muscles, contributing to a more defined waistline.
- Improve rotational mobility and flexibility in the spine, which can decrease the risk of back pain and injury.
- Enhance core stability, which is fundamental for performing daily tasks and other physical activities with ease and less fatigue.
- Support better posture by strengthening the core muscles, which can often become weakened from prolonged sitting or inactivity.
- Increase functional fitness, making it easier to twist, bend, and move through life's activities with agility and less discomfort.

Wall Clock Reach

The "Wall Clock Reach" is a refined exercise within the Wall Pilates Workout regime, tailored specifically for women over 40. This exercise targets several key areas of fitness that are particularly beneficial for this age group, including flexibility, balance, core strength, and the engagement of shoulder muscles. The Wall Clock Reach is not only effective for enhancing physical health but also for improving posture and reducing the risk of injuries by strengthening the muscles around the shoulders and upper back.

Instructions for performing the Wall Clock Reach are as follows:
1. Begin by standing with your right side facing the wall, approximately an arm's length away. Plant your feet firmly on the ground, hip-width apart.
2. Extend your right arm and place your right palm flat against the wall at shoulder height, imagining the wall as the face of a clock.
3. Keeping your arm straight and your palm pressed firmly against the wall, slowly move your hand in a clockwise direction as if tracing the numbers on a clock face. Reach as far as you can while maintaining a flat palm and straight arm, moving from the 12 o'clock position down to 6 o'clock, and back up to 12 o'clock.
4. Once you complete the circle in a clockwise direction, repeat the movement in a counter-clockwise direction, starting from 12 o'clock, moving up to 6 o'clock (above your head), and then back down.

5. Switch sides and repeat the exercise with your left arm, standing with your left side facing the wall.

The benefits of the Wall Clock Reach are multifaceted:

- Improves Shoulder Mobility and Flexibility: This exercise stretches the shoulder muscles, enhancing range of motion and flexibility, which is crucial for preventing stiffness and injuries, especially in the rotator cuff area.

- Strengthens Core Muscles: To maintain balance and posture while performing the Wall Clock Reach, the core muscles are engaged, thus strengthening the abdominal and lower back muscles.

- Enhances Postural Stability: Regular practice of this exercise can contribute to better posture by strengthening the upper back muscles and the deltoids, helping to counteract the effects of prolonged sitting or poor posture habits.

- Reduces Injury Risk: By improving flexibility and strength in the shoulder area, the risk of common injuries associated with aging, such as rotator cuff issues, can be significantly reduced.

- Promotes Mind-Body Coordination: The precise movement of tracing the clock requires focus and coordination, promoting a connection between mind and body that is beneficial for overall well-being.

Wall Lateral Flexion

The Wall Lateral Flexion is a pivotal movement in the realm of Wall Pilates, particularly beneficial for women over 40. This exercise focuses on enhancing flexibility and strengthening the muscles along the sides of the body, including the obliques, which play a crucial role in core stability, posture improvement, and overall mobility. By incorporating Wall Lateral Flexion into their Pilates workout, women over 40 can experience a range of benefits that contribute to a healthier, more balanced body and lifestyle.

Instructions for Wall Lateral Flexion:

1. Begin by standing with your right side facing the wall, feet hip-width apart and parallel to each other.
2. Place your right hand on the wall at shoulder height for support.
3. Extend your left arm overhead, reaching towards the ceiling, while keeping your feet firmly planted on the ground.
4. Inhale deeply, and as you exhale, gently lean your torso towards the wall, creating a C-shape with your body. Your left arm should follow the motion, enhancing the stretch along your left side.
5. Keep your hips facing forward and avoid bending forward or backward. The movement should be strictly to the side to target the lateral muscles effectively.

6. Hold the stretch for a few breaths, feeling the extension along your left side from the hip up through the fingertips.

7. Inhale as you gently come back to the starting position.

8. Repeat the movement several times before switching sides to ensure both sides of the body are equally worked.

Benefits of Wall Lateral Flexion:

- Improves Flexibility: Regular practice of this exercise can significantly increase the flexibility of the spine and the lateral muscles of the torso. This is particularly important for women over 40, as flexibility tends to decrease with age.

- Enhances Core Stability: By engaging the obliques and lateral muscles, Wall Lateral Flexion helps to strengthen the core, which is vital for balance, posture, and preventing back pain.

- Promotes Good Posture: Strengthening the side muscles aids in maintaining an upright posture, which can often be compromised by age-related changes or prolonged sitting.

- Increases Lung Capacity: The stretching involved in this exercise opens up the ribcage, allowing for deeper breaths which can increase oxygen intake and improve overall respiratory health.

- Balances Muscle Strength: Focusing on the lateral muscles ensures a balanced strength throughout the torso, helping to prevent muscular imbalances that can lead to pain and injury.

- Reduces Risk of Injury: By improving flexibility and strength in a controlled manner, the risk of injuries related to daily activities or other forms of exercise is reduced.
- Enhances Body Awareness: Engaging in targeted movements like the Wall Lateral Flexion increases body awareness, allowing for more mindful movement and exercise practices.

Wall Hip Openers

The Wall Hip Openers exercise is an integral component of the Wall Pilates Workout, especially designed for women over 40. This exercise focuses on increasing flexibility, reducing stiffness, and enhancing the range of motion in the hips—a common area of tightness and discomfort in many adults. With age, maintaining hip flexibility becomes crucial for performing daily activities smoothly and preventing injuries.

Instructions for Wall Hip Openers:

1. Begin by standing approximately two feet away from a wall, facing it.
2. Place your hands on the wall at shoulder height for stability.
3. Shift your weight to your right leg, keeping it slightly bent at the knee.
4. Lift your left leg and place the outer ankle just above the right knee, creating a figure-four shape with your legs.
5. Gently bend your standing leg and lean your hips back, as if sitting into a chair, while pressing your hands into the wall for balance.
6. Keep your spine long and your chest lifted, avoiding rounding the back. You should feel a gentle stretch in the outer hip of the lifted leg.
7. Hold this position for 15 to 30 seconds, focusing on relaxing into the stretch with each exhale.

8. Slowly straighten the standing leg and return to the starting position.

9. Repeat on the other side, lifting the right leg and placing it over the left knee.

Benefits of Wall Hip Openers:

- Improves Flexibility: Regularly performing hip openers can significantly increase flexibility in the hip joint and the surrounding muscles, which is vital for maintaining a full range of motion as we age.

- Reduces Pain and Stiffness: These exercises can alleviate stiffness and pain in the hips and lower back, common issues for women over 40. By gently stretching the hip flexors, piriformis, and glutes, you can reduce discomfort caused by sitting for long periods or other sedentary activities.

- Enhances Posture and Balance: Hip openers help in correcting posture by realigning the pelvis and hips, leading to better balance and stability. This is crucial for preventing falls and maintaining independence.

- Supports Healthy Spine: By increasing flexibility in the hips, you reduce the strain on the lower back, which can contribute to a healthier spine alignment and decrease the risk of lower back pain.

- Promotes Emotional Release: The hips are often thought of as a storage area for emotional tension. Engaging in hip opening exercises can release this tension, leading to emotional as well as physical relief.

Wall Knee Lifts

Wall Knee Lifts are an excellent exercise within the Wall Pilates Workout, particularly beneficial for women over 40. This exercise focuses on strengthening the core, improving lower body strength, and enhancing balance, making it a key component of a comprehensive Pilates routine. By utilizing the wall as a stabilizing force, Wall Knee Lifts ensure proper alignment and safety, making them suitable for individuals at various fitness levels.

Instructions for Wall Knee Lifts:

1. Start by standing with your back flat against the wall. Ensure your spine is aligned, with your head, shoulders, and hips touching the wall.
2. Place your feet hip-width apart, directly under your hips, for stability.
3. Engage your core muscles by drawing your belly button towards your spine, ensuring your lower back remains in contact with the wall.
4. Slowly lift one knee towards your chest, as high as comfortably possible, while keeping the other leg straight and grounded. Keep your lifted foot flexed.
5. Hold the position for a moment, focusing on engaging the muscles in your core and maintaining balance.
6. Lower the lifted leg back to the starting position with control.

7. Repeat the movement with the opposite leg, alternating between legs for a set number of repetitions.

Benefits of Wall Knee Lifts:

- Core Strengthening: This exercise directly targets the abdominal muscles, helping to build a stronger core. A strong core is essential for improving posture, reducing lower back pain, and performing daily activities more efficiently.
- Balance Improvement: By performing knee lifts, especially with the added stability of the wall, you can improve your balance. This is particularly beneficial as balance tends to decline with age.
- Lower Body Engagement: Although primarily a core exercise, Wall Knee Lifts also engage the muscles in the thighs and glutes. This contributes to lower body strength, which is vital for mobility and joint health.
- Flexibility Increase: Regularly performing knee lifts can increase flexibility in the hip flexors. This is important for maintaining a full range of motion, reducing the risk of injuries, and alleviating stiffness.
- Accessibility: Using the wall for support makes this exercise accessible for those who may have balance concerns or are new to Pilates. It provides a safe way to engage in physical activity without the need for specialized equipment.

Advanced Modifications

How to Increase Intensity

When it comes to enhancing the challenge of a Wall Pilates Workout for women over 40, advancing the intensity of exercises is key for continued physical improvement and maintaining engagement. Here are several strategies for incorporating advanced modifications into a Wall Pilates routine:

1. Incorporate Prop Use: Adding props such as resistance bands, Pilates rings, or stability balls can significantly increase the intensity of wall exercises. For instance, holding a Pilates ring between the hands during wall push-ups adds an extra layer of resistance, engaging the chest and arm muscles more deeply.

2. Adjust Hand and Foot Positions: Simply changing the position of your hands and feet can alter the difficulty level of an exercise. Moving your feet closer to the wall during exercises like the wall plank or wall sit decreases stability, forcing your muscles to work harder to maintain balance and form.

3. Increase Range of Motion: Extending the range of motion in exercises like the wall roll-down or wall leg lifts challenges your flexibility and strength further. Try reaching lower or lifting higher, always ensuring

movements are controlled and within comfortable limits to avoid strain.

4. Add Movement Complexity: Introducing additional movements into a basic exercise can significantly increase its intensity. For example, incorporating leg lifts or knee tucks during a wall plank not only engages the core more intensively but also involves the lower body, enhancing the overall challenge.

5. Elevate Repetition and Sets: Increasing the number of repetitions and sets is a straightforward approach to intensify any workout. If the original routine calls for 10 wall squats, pushing it to 15 or 20 repetitions adds more endurance training to the session.

6. Shorten Rest Periods: Decreasing the amount of rest time between exercises keeps the heart rate elevated, adds a cardiovascular component to the strength training, and makes the workout more challenging. This approach should be used cautiously, ensuring enough rest to maintain proper form throughout.

7. Incorporate Isometric Holds: Adding holds to exercises, such as pausing at the lowest point of a wall squat or holding the peak of a wall push-up, increases muscle tension and endurance. These isometric holds can be incorporated before completing the movement to add an extra challenge.

Advanced Variations for Core Exercises

Incorporating advanced variations into core exercises can significantly enhance the effectiveness of a Wall Pilates workout for women over 40. These modifications are designed to challenge the body further, increasing strength, stability, and flexibility in the core, which is vital for overall health and well-being. By introducing more complex movements and adding resistance, these advanced variations can help deepen the Pilates practice.

One advanced variation is the elevated feet wall plank. By placing the feet on the wall at a higher position while in a plank, the gravitational pull increases the intensity of the core engagement. This position demands more stability and strength from the abdominal muscles, the obliques, and the lower back, enhancing the traditional plank's benefits.

Another variation involves incorporating leg movements into the wall bridge. Once in the bridge position with the feet pressed against the wall, alternately extending one leg at a time increases the challenge. This not only tests the strength of the glutes and hamstrings but also requires the core to work harder to maintain stability and balance.

For those looking to intensify their workout further, adding a twist to the wall sit can engage the obliques more deeply. While in a wall sit position, rotating the torso to one side with the arms extended, then alternating sides, can add a dynamic element to the isometric exercise. This movement not only strengthens the core but also enhances rotational mobility.

Incorporating a Pilates ball between the wall and the lower back during wall squats introduces instability, forcing the core to engage more deeply to maintain balance. As the squat is performed, the ball rolls slightly up and down the wall, requiring constant adjustments from the core muscles to perform the movement smoothly.

For a more challenging version of the wall push-up, one can experiment with an asymmetrical hand position. Placing one hand higher on the wall and the other lower shifts the focus and intensity of the exercise, engaging the core muscles differently on each side. This variation not only strengthens the upper body but also encourages the core to stabilize the body against the uneven forces.

Transitioning from wall exercises to floor exercises near the wall can also add variety and intensity. For example, performing a supine leg drop with the legs elevated against the wall targets the lower abdominals. Lowering the legs toward the ground without touching it, then raising them back up, challenges the core's strength and endurance.

Lastly, integrating resistance bands into wall Pilates exercises can introduce a new level of difficulty. Attaching a band to a stable point or closing it in a door, then using it for exercises like the standing twist or the side pull, adds resistance that the core must work against. This not only strengthens the muscles but also enhances proprioception and coordination.

These advanced variations are designed to push the limits of what the body can achieve, particularly for women over 40 who are looking to deepen their Pilates practice. As always, it's important to listen to the body and consult with a healthcare provider before attempting more challenging exercises, especially if there are any existing health concerns.

Challenging Upper and Lower Body Combinations

In the realm of Wall Pilates, particularly for women over 40, advancing one's practice through challenging upper and lower body combinations can lead to significant gains in strength, flexibility, and overall fitness. These advanced modifications are designed to provide a comprehensive workout that tests and improves endurance, balance, and core stability, all while being mindful of the unique needs of this age group.

One dynamic combination involves integrating the Wall Plank with Leg Lifts. This exercise challenges the core, shoulders, and glutes simultaneously. By facing the wall, placing hands at shoulder height, and extending one leg at a time while maintaining a plank position, the practitioner engages multiple muscle groups. This not only builds upper body strength but also enhances balance and coordination, crucial for maintaining functional fitness.

Transitioning to the Wall Squat with Heel Raises adds an element of lower body endurance and calf strengthening to the routine. Performing a squat against the wall and then lifting the heels while maintaining the squat position targets the quadriceps, hamstrings, and calves. This exercise emphasizes stability and control, engaging the core and lower back muscles to support posture and alignment.

For a more intense upper body challenge, Wall Push-Ups can be adapted by altering hand positions or adding a single-leg lift. These modifications increase the difficulty by requiring more strength and balance, engaging the chest, triceps, and core muscles more deeply. Such variations can enhance muscular endurance and promote upper body toning.

Incorporating the Wall Teaser involves using the wall as support to perform a V-sit, which intensely activates the abdominal muscles and hip flexors, while also challenging the balance and stability of the lower back. This exercise is a testament to the adaptability of Pilates principles, bringing a classic Pilates exercise to the wall for added support and depth.

To challenge the lower body further, the Wall Bridge with Single-Leg Extension tests the glutes, hamstrings, and core. Lying on the ground with feet pressed against the wall, lifting into a bridge position, and then extending one leg at a time into the air increases the intensity of the workout, fostering muscular strength and endurance in the lower body.

An advanced combination that targets both the upper and lower body is the Wall Side Plank with Leg Lifts. This exercise requires side-facing the wall, placing one hand on the wall, lifting into a side plank, and then raising the top leg. It's a comprehensive movement that strengthens the obliques, shoulders, and outer thighs, contributing to improved side-body strength and balance.

For women over 40 looking to elevate their Wall Pilates practice, these advanced modifications offer a pathway to enhanced physical health and vitality. They represent a balanced approach to fitness, combining strength, flexibility, and balance training in a way that respects the body's needs and limitations. By progressively challenging themselves with these exercises, practitioners can experience marked improvements in their Pilates practice, leading to greater well-being and a more active lifestyle.

Practice Schedule

Suggested Weekly Routine

Crafting a weekly routine for Wall Pilates workouts tailored for women over 40 involves balancing exercise with rest, ensuring a holistic approach to fitness that promotes strength, flexibility, and well-being while minimizing the risk of injury. Given the unique needs and considerations of this age group, including the increased need for warm-up time and recovery, a thoughtful schedule is key to maximizing the benefits of Wall Pilates.

A suggested weekly routine could begin on Monday with a focus on core and stability exercises. This might include movements such as Wall Planks, Wall Sit, and Wall Roll-Downs to engage the core muscles thoroughly, setting a strong foundation for the week's activities. Core strength is vital for posture, balance, and overall fitness, making it an excellent starting point.

On Tuesday, the routine could shift to emphasize upper body strength and flexibility. Exercises like Wall Push-Ups, Triceps Push-Up With Side Leg Lift, and Wall Arm Circles can target the arms, shoulders, and upper back. This day should also incorporate stretches such as the Wall Chest Opener to ensure muscles remain flexible and to reduce the risk of tension buildup.

Wednesday could serve as a day for focusing on lower body strength and endurance. Incorporating Wall Squats, Single-Leg Bridge With Abduction, and Wall Reverse Lunges can target the legs and glutes, areas that are crucial for mobility and daily activities. Stretching exercises like the Wall Hamstring Stretch and Wall Calf Stretch would be beneficial to conclude the session, aiding in muscle recovery and flexibility.

Thursday could be a designated rest day or a light activity day. Given the importance of recovery, especially for women over 40, engaging in gentle yoga, a leisurely walk, or a restorative Pilates session without the wall could help maintain activity levels without overexerting muscles. This day is crucial for allowing the body to recover and rebuild.

On Friday, the routine could combine elements from the week's workouts, focusing on full-body integration. This might include a circuit of selected exercises from the previous days or introducing dynamic movements like the Wall Bicycle and Wall Side Leg Lifts that engage multiple muscle groups simultaneously. The goal is to reinforce the week's work by engaging the entire body in a cohesive manner.

Saturday's routine could focus on balance and agility, incorporating exercises like the Wall Clock Reach and Wall Oblique Twist. These movements challenge the body's balance and coordination, which are essential for overall fitness and injury prevention. Ending the session with deep breathing exercises and wall-supported stretches can promote relaxation and flexibility.

Sunday, then, should be a day of rest or very gentle activity, emphasizing the importance of rest in any fitness regimen. This day is for allowing the body to fully recover, ensuring that muscles have time to repair and strengthen. Engaging in mindfulness practices, such as meditation or gentle stretching, can also support mental well-being, rounding out the holistic approach to fitness.

This weekly routine is just a suggestion and should be adapted based on individual fitness levels, health considerations, and personal goals. It's always recommended to consult with a fitness professional or healthcare provider before starting any new exercise program, especially for those with pre-existing health conditions or those who are new to physical activity.

How to Progress

Progressing in a Wall Pilates Workout for women over 40 involves a thoughtful approach that balances challenge with safety, ensuring a gradual improvement in strength, flexibility, and overall well-being. The key to advancing in your practice is to systematically increase the intensity and complexity of exercises while incorporating principles of mindfulness and body awareness.

At the outset, it's crucial to establish a consistent routine. Beginning with three sessions a week allows the body to adapt to the new physical demands without overwhelming it. Each session should start with a comprehensive warm-up to prepare the muscles and joints, followed by a series of foundational exercises that focus on core strength, balance, and flexibility. Over time, the frequency of these workouts can be increased, but it's essential to listen to the body and allow for adequate rest.

As comfort with the basic movements grows, the next step is to gradually introduce more advanced exercises or increase the number of repetitions for each exercise. It's not just about doing more; it's about doing better. Paying attention to form and technique ensures that each movement is as effective as possible. This attention to detail can make even familiar exercises more challenging and beneficial.

Another way to progress is by incorporating variations of standard exercises to challenge different muscle groups. For example, modifying the wall push-up by altering hand placement can target the chest and arms differently. Similarly, adding leg lifts or squats before coming into a wall sit can increase lower body strength and endurance.

Adding small equipment like resistance bands or Pilates balls can also introduce a new level of resistance, making the exercises more challenging. These tools can help deepen the engagement of specific muscles and add variety to the workout, keeping it interesting and engaging as you progress.

Setting personal goals can be a powerful motivator. Whether it's improving posture, enhancing flexibility, or increasing core strength, having clear objectives can guide the progression of the workout routine. Periodically revisiting these goals and celebrating achievements, no matter how small, can provide a sense of accomplishment and encourage continued effort.

Finally, integrating principles of mindfulness and deep breathing into each session can enhance the connection between mind and body, a core aspect of Pilates. As physical capabilities grow, so too should the focus on breath control and mental clarity. This holistic approach ensures that progression in wall Pilates is not just about physical achievements but also about fostering a sense of well-being and inner strength.

By following these guidelines, women over 40 can safely and effectively progress in their wall Pilates workouts, enjoying the benefits of improved physical health and a greater sense of balance and vitality in their lives.

Adjusting the Routine to Your Fitness Level

Adjusting a Wall Pilates workout routine to match one's fitness level is crucial, particularly for women over 40, who may have diverse health and fitness backgrounds. Tailoring your Pilates practice ensures that the exercises are both challenging and achievable, minimizing the risk of injury while maximizing benefits. This personalized approach encourages consistency and progression, leading to more significant long-term health improvements.

For beginners or those who are returning to exercise after a period of inactivity, starting with the basics is key. Focus on mastering the form of each exercise, such as wall squats, wall push-ups, and gentle stretches like the wall-supported cat-cow. Begin with fewer repetitions, paying close attention to how your body feels during and after each exercise. It's more beneficial to perform a smaller number of exercises correctly than to rush through a routine without proper form.

As your strength and confidence grow, gradually increase the intensity of your workouts. This could mean adding more repetitions, incorporating more challenging exercises such as the wall plank or wall pike, or holding positions like the wall sit for longer periods. The beauty of Wall Pilates is the ease with which you can adjust the difficulty level. Simply altering the angle of your body against the wall or increasing the duration of each exercise can significantly enhance the challenge.

Listening to your body is paramount. If a particular movement feels too strenuous, modify it or choose an alternative that targets the same muscle group. For instance, if a full wall plank is too challenging, adjust by moving your feet closer to the wall to reduce the angle and decrease the intensity. This flexibility in modifying exercises ensures that you can continue working out even on days when you might not feel at your best.

Incorporating rest days into your routine is also essential. Pilates, while low-impact, still exerts stress on the muscles and joints. Women over 40 should allow adequate recovery time between sessions to prevent overuse injuries and ensure muscles have time to repair and strengthen. A balanced routine might include Wall Pilates exercises three to four times a week, interspersed with rest or active recovery days featuring lighter activities like walking or yoga.

Varying your routine can help prevent plateaus and maintain motivation. After a few weeks of consistent practice, introduce new exercises or variations to keep the workouts interesting and challenging. This not only helps to improve overall fitness but also ensures that all muscle groups are engaged and strengthened over time.

Finally, setting realistic goals and tracking progress can be highly motivating. Whether it's improving flexibility, increasing strength, or enhancing balance, having clear objectives can guide the adjustment of your workout routine to better align with your fitness level and aspirations. Celebrating small victories along the way fosters a positive relationship with exercise and encourages long-term commitment to a healthy lifestyle.

Adjusting a Wall Pilates routine for women over 40 involves starting slowly, progressively increasing intensity, modifying exercises as needed, incorporating rest days, varying the routine, and setting realistic goals. This thoughtful approach ensures that Pilates remains a safe, enjoyable, and effective workout option for women seeking to enhance their fitness at any age.

Conclusion

Beginning on the Wall Pilates Workout adventure for women over 40 is more than just doing a set of exercises; it is about beginning on a transforming journey that benefits both the body and mind. This journey, designed expressly for the unique needs and talents of women at this lively stage of life, concludes with a profound appreciation for what our bodies can accomplish with care, respect, and devotion.

As we wrap up our examination of Wall Pilates, it's important to reflect on our development. The path has most certainly included hardships, moments of self-doubt, and maybe even times of stagnation. However, it has also provided moments of success, more self-awareness, and increased confidence in one's physical talents. The beauty of Wall Pilates is not just the physical strength acquired, but also the mental resilience and clarity developed through constant practice.

The dedication to incorporating Wall Pilates into one's lifestyle goes beyond physical health. It is a dedication to promoting one's own well-being, acknowledging the body's desire for movement, and recognizing its limitations. Wall Pilates is a haven for women over 40 who are typically juggling professions, families, and personal growth. It enhances not just their muscles, but also their determination and focus.

One of the most essential lessons learned on this trip is the need of adaptation and patience. Wall Pilates teaches us to listen to our bodies, alter routines as necessary, and celebrate tiny triumphs along the way. This technique promotes a gentle yet meaningful approach to fitness that ideally suits the demands of women navigating the challenges of life beyond 40.

Looking ahead, the trip does not finish here. The ideas and movements of Wall Pilates form the basis for a lifetime of health and fitness. The practice's versatility allows it to evolve alongside you, providing new challenges and chances for growth as your requirements and skills change. This constant progress is what distinguishes Wall Pilates as a lifestyle rather than just a workout.

For women over 40, the Wall Pilates Workout is more than simply a physical fitness instruction; it's an invitation to a journey of self-discovery, empowerment, and overall wellness. It demonstrates that women of any age may reinvent their connection with their bodies by embracing strength, flexibility, and balance, both physically and emotionally.

To summarize, the Wall Pilates Workout for Women Over 40 is about more than just finishing a fitness program; it is about continuing a path of personal growth, health, and well-being. It is about bringing the lessons taught, the strength acquired, and the confidence developed into all aspects of life. It celebrates what it means to be a woman over 40 today: strong, adaptive, and undeniably energetic.

28-Days Workout Program

Day	Focus Area	Exercise	Duration	Notes
1	Core & Balance	Wall Standing Pilates	10 mins	Focus on breathing and posture
2	Legs & Glutes	Wall Squats	10 mins	Keep back flat against the wall
3	Rest & Recover	-	-	Focus on stretching or a light walk
4	Arms & Shoulders	Wall Push-Ups	10 mins	Elbows at a 45-degree angle
5	Core & Flexibility	Wall Plank	5 mins	Increase time as it becomes easier
6	Full Body	Wall Sit & Stretch	15 mins	Combine squats with stretching intervals
7	Rest & Recover	-	-	Optional gentle yoga or meditation

Day	Focus Area	Exercise	Duration	Notes
8	Core & Balance	Wall Leg Raises	10 mins	Increase reps as comfortable
9	Legs & Glutes	Wall Lunge	10 mins	Maintain alignment of knee and ankle
10	Rest & Recover	-	-	Focus on hydration and nutrition
11	Arms & Shoulders	Wall Side Plank	10 mins	Switch sides for balance
12	Core & Flexibility	Wall Bridge	10 mins	Press lower back into the wall
13	Full Body	Wall Pilates Flow	15 mins	Sequence of previous exercises
14	Rest & Recover	-	-	Consider a massage or self-care activity
15	Core & Balance	Wall V-Sit	10 mins	Adjust angle for difficulty
16	Legs & Glutes	Wall Calf Raises	10 mins	Use wall for balance

Day	Focus Area	Exercise	Duration	Notes
17	Rest & Recover	-	-	Light stretching or foam rolling
18	Arms & Shoulders	Wall Tricep Dips	10 mins	Chair or low wall needed
19	Core & Flexibility	Wall Twist	10 mins	Focus on obliques
20	Full Body	Wall Pilates Series	20 mins	Integrate all muscle group exercises
21	Rest & Recover	-	-	Relaxation techniques or light walk
22	Core & Balance	Wall Scissor Kicks	10 mins	Engage core throughout
23	Legs & Glutes	Wall Pelvic Tilts	10 mins	Focus on pelvic floor muscles
24	Rest & Recover	-	-	Stay hydrated and eat well

Day	Focus Area	Exercise	Duration	Notes
25	Arms & Shoulders	Wall Circle Arms	10 mins	Improve shoulder mobility
26	Core & Flexibility	Wall Pike	10 mins	Adjust difficulty by feet placement
27	Full Body	Wall Pilates Challenge	20 mins	Combine exercises in a flowing sequence
28	Rest, Reflect, & Celebrate	-	-	Reflect on progress and plan ahead